Benjamin Bryan

Anti-Vivisection Evidences

A collection of authentic statements by competent witnesses as to the immorality,

cruelty, and futility of experiments on living animals

Benjamin Bryan

Anti-Vivisection Evidences
A collection of authentic statements by competent witnesses as to the immorality, cruelty, and futility of experiments on living animals

ISBN/EAN: 9783337241452

Printed in Europe, USA, Canada, Australia, Japan

Cover: Foto ©Suzi / pixelio.de

More available books at **www.hansebooks.com**

ANTI-VIVISECTION EVIDENCES.

A COLLECTION

OF

Authentic Statements by Competent Witnesses

AS TO THE

IMMORALITY, CRUELTY, AND FUTILITY

OF

EXPERIMENTS ON LIVING ANIMALS.

By BENJAMIN BRYAN.

NEW EDITION, REVISED AND ENLARGED.

ABBREVIATIONS:

A.V. Anti-Vivisectionist.
R. Restrictionist.
V. Vivisector or Vivisectionist.
P.V. Pro-Vivisectionist.
N. Neutral.

LONDON:
SOCIETY FOR THE PROTECTION OF ANIMALS FROM
VIVISECTION, 20, VICTORIA STREET, S.W.
1895
Price Six Shillings.

PREFACE.

SCATTERED up and down in different places there are a great number of Evidences against Vivisection; but their value has hitherto been greatly diminished through their having been so scattered. This book represents an attempt to collect and arrange them in order for speedy reference. The collection is not and does not profess to be exhaustive; but even in its present form it is hoped it may be found useful. The whole of the extracts are authentic, and are verified by having their sources fully shown; an index to authors has also been added, which it is hoped will still further enhance the value of the book.

B. B.

May, 1895.

ANTI-VIVISECTION EVIDENCES.

ABNORMAL CONDITION of Vivisected Animals.   Richet.

CHARLES RICHET, M.D., Professor of Physiology, Faculty of Medicine, Paris. (V.)

" Pain is a purely central phenomenon. It is a sensation that may exist, even to intensity, without manifesting its presence by any external sign, and consequently it is impossible to gauge it. All physiologists know that during vivisection there is an entire dissimilarity in the manner in which animals seem to suffer. Some remain motionless, the eyes fixed, neither struggling nor moaning ; they appear as if struck by stupor. Others, on the contrary, groan and howl, never remaining a moment without struggling or endeavouring to escape. Every incision that is made, every laceration, every pull is instantly followed by a shock which interferes with the result of the experiment. . . . I will point out, moreover, the fact observed by the physiologists at Alfort. The blood of the animals used for operations is almost devoid of fibrin, like the blood of animals that have been overworked. As regards dyspepsia and disorders of the digestive functions which prolonged pain brings on, the phenomenon is rather psychical than physiological, and pain acts similarly to grief and privation."—" *Recherches Expérimentelles et Cliniques sur la Sensibilité*," *Collection de Thèses, Ecole de Médicine* (Paris, 1877), p. 255.

—— The same.   Fergusson.

SIR WILLIAM FERGUSSON, F.R.S. (the late), Sergeant-Surgeon to the Queen. (Born 1808 ; died 1877.) (A.V.)

" I do not think, referring to the most recent experiments that have been made, that you can form a very accurate opinion as to the actions of nature from looking through the walls of the abdomen at the liver. You get a window cut in the side of the abdomen, and get the gall bladder laid open, and you look at it

B

or a physiologist looks at it, and watches it a certain number
of hours or days; but the animal is put into such an extra-
ordinary condition by all that has been done, that I cannot say
that I have very great confidence in the results of such an
experiment. . . . A great distinction should be drawn
between the two, I think. Very often certain operations are
performed on the lower animals, and these experiments are
used in a way that they never would be used in the human
subject."—*Evid. Roy. Com.* (London, 1876), Q. 1051-2.

ABNORMAL CONDITION of Vivisected   Macaulay.
Animals.

JAMES MACAULAY, M.A., M.D., F.R.C.S.Ed., London. (A.V.)

"That observations made by vivisection are of necessity
abnormal and liable to fallacy, reason alone might show, independently of experience. The sources of error arise, not from
any contingent cause, but from the very nature of this method
of investigation. Nature, when interrogated, reveals only what
is her condition at the moment of examination ; and hence,
although the permanent and unvarying properties of inanimate
matter render the use of experiment of paramount value, the
questioning process is more limited, and its results more uncertain, when applied to living and sentient beings. We cannot
depend on the accuracy of conclusions respecting the normal
functions of parts, if drawn from experiments which only tell
what takes place in those unnatural conditions induced by
operations. For not only are the ordinary actions of the organs
thereby often deranged or destroyed, but many causes conspire
to render still wider the difference between the observed and
the natural condition of the subjects operated upon. The
deadening of pain during the actual use of the knife and other
instruments,is only one element in the contrast,although chloroform itself in many cases increases the sources of fallacy and
interferes with results. The excitement and terror of the animal
must be taken into account ; and there is abnormal action, even
if the body be made insensible and unconscious."—"*Vivisection,*"
A Prize Essay (London, 1881), pp. 61-62.

ABOLITION, Arguments for.   Swan.

WILLIAM SWAN, LL.D., Edin., and St. Andrew ; Emeritus
Professor of Natural Philosophy in the University of St. Andrew's.
(A.V.)

"Striking the balance between good and evil *now* done by
vivisection, we may assuredly say, in familiar phrase, ' the game

is not worth the candle.' If, then, we cannot obtain the legislative prohibition of vivisection for mere educational purposes, along with its very rigorous restriction in cases of physiological research, I, for one, would say—' Better put an end to the practice *absolutely*, without any exceptions whatever.' I will add but a word as to the claims for effectual protection of the poor defenceless animals so ruthlessly tormented. Their cry for compassionate sympathy cannot fail to find an echo in every true heart."—*Letter to Mrs. Watson, of Edinburgh*, 1891.

ABUSE OF VIVISECTION, Liability to. Royal Commission.

FROM THE REPORT OF THE ROYAL COMMISSION.
(London : Eyre and Spottiswoode, 1876.)

"We find that until a comparatively recent period physiology . . . had been for some time past but little cultivated in this country, but that there has been of late years a great movement in advance. . . . There is at the present time . . . a great scientific revival (page vii). *[Increase of Physiology.]*

" We think it most desirable that an effectual restraint should be placed upon what Dr. Taylor has described to us as purposeless cruelty ; on experiments made in excessive numbers ; on experiments made to establish what has been already proved ; on experiments attended with great pain, and defeating the very object in view ; on experiments made where a man has been desirous of bringing himself forward, or trying a new thing merely for the sake of a little notoriety. . . . (page xiv). *[Restraint on purposeless cruelty.]*

"Sir Thomas Watson, Sir George Burrows, Sir James Paget, and many others have suggested the analogy of the Anatomy Act (for legislation) and some scientific witnesses have expressed their opinion that the interference of the legislature is called for in the interests, not only of humanity, but also of science. Sir William Fergusson thinks that if the public really knew what was actually going on in this country at this time, they would expect an interference on the part of the Crown and Parliament, just as much as with reference to the disinterring of dead bodies years ago. . . . (page xv). *[Public, if they knew all, would expect interference.]*

Called on to recommend legislation.

" But even if the weight of authority on the side of legislative interference had been less considerable, we should have thought ourselves called upon *Practice liable to great abuse.* to recommend it by the reason of the thing. It is manifest that the practice is from its very nature *Inhumanity in* liable to great abuse. . . . It is not to be *persons highly placed.* doubted that inhumanity may be found in persons of very high positions as physiologists. . . . We *Students have tortured animals.* have had some evidence that cases have arisen in which the unpractised student has taken upon himself without guidance in his private lodgings to expose animals to torture without anæsthetics for no purpose which could merit the name of legitimate scientific research. Evidence of this nature is not easily obtained. . . . Besides the cases in which inhumanity exists, we are satis- *Carelessness and indifference.* fied there are others in which carelessness and indifference prevail to an extent sufficient to form a ground for legislative interference . . . we have been much struck by the consideration that *Severe experiments for in-adequate results.* severe experiments have been engaged in for the purpose of establishing results which have been considered inadequate to justify that severity, by persons of very competent authority (page xvii).

Experiments to be under control.

" What we should humbly recommend to your Majesty would be the enactment of a law by which experiments upon living animals, whether for original research or for demonstration, should be placed under the control of the Secretary of State, who should have power to grant licences and . . . to withdraw them. . . . (page xx).

Efficient in-spection.

" The Secretary of State must have the most complete powers of efficient inspection. . . . The Inspectors must be persons of such character and position as to command the confidence of the public, no less than that of men of science. . . . *All this com-patible with medical pro-gress.* We believe that by such a measure as we have now proposed the progress of medical knowledge may be made compatible with the just requirements *Claim of lower animals to be humanely treated to be recognised.* of humanity. . . . We trust that Your Majesty's Government and the Parliament of this kingdom will recognise the claim of the lower animals to be treated with humane consideration, and will establish the right of the community to be assured that this claim shall not be forgotten amid the triumphs of advancing science.

"(Signed)   CARDWELL.
                WINMARLEIGH.
                W. E. FORSTER.
                JOHN B. KARSLAKE.
                T. H. HUXLEY.
                JOHN ERIC ERICHSEN.
—(page xxi)   RICHARD HOLT HUTTON."

ACONITINA (MONKSHOOD), Contradictory   Berdoe. Results of Experiments with.

EDWARD BERDOE, M.R.C.S., L.R.C.P.Ed., London. (A.V.)

"Achscharumow says that in frogs aconitina produces at first a reduction in the number of the heart's pulsations, then an increase in the rapidity of its action.—(*Reichert's Archiv*, 1866, p. 255.)

"Achscharumow argues that the slowing of the pulse during the early stage of aconite-poisoning is due to the stimulation of the inhibiting centres in the medulla oblongata.—(p. 272.)

"The most diverse conclusions have been arrived at by different vivisectors as to the action of aconitina upon the nervous system. Achscharumow says that the spinal cord is not affected.—(*Wood*, p. 174.)

"Lauder-Brunton says : 'The heart in the frog is first quickened and then slowed. In man or mammals there is first slowness of the pulse, but shortly before death it may become more rapid.'—(*Pharmacology*, p. 750.)

"Böhm and Wartman repudiate this conclusion.—(*Loc. cit.*, p. 266.)

"Later investigations have, however, clearly shown that some fallacy exists in the studies of Achscharumow.—(*Wood*, p. 174.)

"Lauder-Brunton says (p. 750): 'The motor centres of the spinal cord, and the respiratory and vaso-motor centres in the medulla, appear first to be slightly stimulated, so that clonic convulsions may occur. The reflex power of the cord is diminished.'"—*The Futility of Experiments with Drugs on Animals.* By Edward Berdoe (London, 1889), pp. 6–7.

See *also* DRUGS, for the pain caused by experiments with Aconite.

ACT, The, Summary of.   39 and 40 Vict. ch. 77.

Clause 1.—Short title, "The Cruelty to Animals Act, 1876."

Clause 2.—Prohibits any painful experiment on a living animal (except subject to certain restrictions explained later on in the Act), and provides a penalty of £50 for the first (and £100 or three months' imprisonment for any subsequent) offence for any person taking part in such experiment.

Clause 3.—Explains the restrictions, which are: (1) The experiment must be performed to advance new physiological discoveries, or knowledge useful in prolonging life or alleviating suffering. (2) The experimenter must hold a licence from the Secretary of State, and, in case of holders of conditional certificates, may only perform the experiments in registered places. (3 and 4) The animal must be under the influence of an anæsthetic of sufficient power to prevent pain throughout the experiment ; and if pain be likely to follow, the animal must be killed before recovering from the anæsthetic. (5 and 6) The experiments may not be performed as illustrative of lectures in medical schools, etc., nor for the purpose of attaining manual skill. Certain provisos follow, which permit (subject in each case to a special certificate being obtained from the Home Secretary by the experimenter): (1) That experiments with anæsthetics may be used for illustrations of lectures to students, if absolutely necessary for their instruction. (2 and 3) That where the use of anæsthetics would frustrate the object of the experiment, they may be dispensed with during its progress, and as long after as it is necessary, provided the animal be killed when the object is attained. (4) Experiments not necessarily for new discoveries, but for testing former ones, if such be "absolutely necessary," for the effectual advancement of such knowledge.

Clause 4.—Explains that urari, or curare, shall not be deemed an anæsthetic. (Its use is not interfered with.)

Clause 5.—Prohibits (except by certificate—to be granted by the Home Secretary) painful experiments on dogs and cats without anæsthetics, and any painful experiments on horses, asses, or mules, unless the object of such experiment would be frustrated by substituting any other animal.

Clause 6.—Absolutely prohibits any experiment upon a living animal in public, and provides penalties to all concerned in such offence.

ADMINISTRATION OF LAW.

Clause 7.—Permits the Secretary of State to make the registration of the place for the proposed experiments a condition of granting the license, provided he approves of the place.

Clause 8.—Permits the Secretary of State to grant a license to any person he deems qualified : gives him power to revoke any license, or to annex any conditions to it for the better carrying into effect the objects of the Act.

Clause 9.—Permits the Secretary of State to call for reports of experiments, with such details as he may require.

Clause 10.—Provides for the inspection from time to time of all licensed places, "for the purpose of securing a compliance with the provisions of this Act."

Clause 11.—Gives a list of the presidents of learned societies and others, whose endorsement must be obtained by any applicant for a license, or certificate under this Act.

Clause 12.—Permits a judge to issue a license for experiment upon living animals, if necessary for evidence, in criminal cases.

Legal Proceedings.

Clause 13.—Permits entry into unlicensed places upon suspicion, under a warrant obtained (according to certain formalities) from a justice of the peace. and provides penalties for obstruction.

Clause 14.—Recommends the prosecution of such offenders under the Summary Jurisdiction Act, and defines the court.

Clause 15.—Allows the accused in England to object to being tried by a Court of Summary Jurisdiction, and in such case permits the court to remit the case for trial as an indictable offence.

Clause 16.—Explains the method of appeal from the foregoing courts.

Clause 17.—Defines the legal proceedings for Scotland.

Clauses 18, 19, and 20.—Define the legal proceedings for Ireland.

Clause 21.—Permits the prosecution of a licensed person, only by the written assent of the Secretary of State.

Clause 22.—Excludes invertebrate animals from the operation of the Act.

ACT, The, Interpreted.   Coleridge.

HON. BERNARD (now LORD) COLERIDGE, Q.C., M.P., London. (A.V.)

This Act "which is something of a compromise on the face of it," no doubt limits the practice of vivisection to some extent. Prior to the Act, any one could vivisect any animal, other than a domestic animal, with or without anæsthetics, where, how. and when he pleased. This unlimited vivisection is now illegal.

The restrictions, however, imposed by Clause 3 in its first

group of six sub-clauses, had they gone further and "prohibited all vivisection save in a registered place, and in the presence of an inspector," would then have indeed limited, as the Act professes to limit, the infliction of pain upon animals.

"But the Act does not complete these restrictions by such an addition," nor does it even leave them where they stand, but "immediately over-rides them by a series of provisos which deliver over the animals to the will and pleasure of holders of licenses and certificates." These permits are issued at the discretion of the Secretary of State, upon certain applications being presented signed by those who are most probably them-selves vivisectors.

The simple license holder who has no certificate is bound by these restrictions, but there is no machinery provided by the Act to guarantee their observance. No inspector can intrude upon him, nor can a constable upon a warrant obtained from a Justice of Peace (see Section 13) intrude upon the premises of a holder of a licence. "In vain might his neighbour on oath state to a justice that, having heard the cries of animals in pain, he had reason to believe that anæsthetics were not being administered, in spite of the fact that the vivisector held no certificate authorising him to dispense with their use," the answer would be that, as he held a license, although the belief of the informer might be well founded, "an Englishman's home is his castle."

The Secretary of State *may* insert (Clause 7) as a condition of granting a license, a provision that the place where any experiment is to be performed is to be registered. But for him to do this is purely optional. Even if he insert it (according to Clause 10), "There is no provision that the inspector shall be there during the performance of the experiment;" nor any "compulsory notice to be given by the operator to the inspector of the time at which the operation is to be performed." A minute inspection of the lavatory, vivisection trough, and instruments, *when the operator was not performing an operation*, would do nothing to secure compliance to the Act.

Such is the position of the holder of the simple license, whose identity (like that of the holders of certificates which give such scope for vivisection) is shrouded in mystery. There is no pro-vision by which the public may know who hold them. The certificates which override the restrictions allow, in the first place : vivisection to be practised by way of illustrations of lectures, the object of which is to advance physiological knowledge wholly unconnected with any useful and humane purpose.

In the next place, it is an open question whether the holder of a certificate under the 1st proviso may not go further, and, with a certificate obtained under the 2nd or 3rd proviso, operate by way of illustration to lectures without an anæsthetic, or if that be used, without obligation to kill before the animal has recovered from its influence. Probably the Act intended all operations illustrating lectures to be performed under anæsthetics and with the obligation to kill. But has it said so ? A Penal Act is to be construed most strictly in favour of the accused : so although the fifth restriction prohibits experiments as illustrations to lectures, and the only proviso enlarging it provides that anæsthetics must be used, yet certificates granted under Provisos 2 and 3 are general and unqualified in their terms.

Again, there is nothing to prevent a vivisector who holds a certificate signed by A. and B., providing himself with another dispensing with anæsthetics, signed by C. and D. Doctors proverbially differ. Not only is there the difficulty of applying an anæsthetic thoroughly and regulating its force and duration : but there are experiments where a vivid sensation (a lively feeling of agony) is essential to the desired object, which would be frustrated by its use.

Armed with a certificate under Proviso 2, there is no limit to the acuteness or continuance of the pain which a vivisector may inflict. If he also hold one under Proviso 4, he may use it to test a former discovery. This permits of the enormous proportion of experiments in this class, undertaken for the mere purposes of controversy.

Proviso 3, dispensing with the necessity of killing, admits of the performance of experiments involving protracted agony.

Holders of certificates may by law inflict upon animals the severest cruelties of which the mind of man can conceive. Nor does the Act place any limit to the number of animals that may be sacrificed, whether under a license or a certificate.

The intending vivisector will find among the list of those enumerated as empowered to sign his certificate a large number " who hold all the opinions ascribed to those who approve of vivisection."

Although curare is held to prevent all muscular movement, it does not prevent but rather increases the feeling of pain. Its use is here made perfectly lawful. The simple licensee may use it in conjunction with an anæsthetic ; and when the effect of the anæsthetic has passed away, leaving the animal still under the influence of the drug, which makes it conveniently silent and motionless, who shall correct his statements ? It is impracticable in a paralysed and motionless creature to ascertain when an anæsthetic takes effect. Thus curare makes anæsthetics useless.

The holder of a certificate dispensing with the use of anæsthetics may use this terrible substance at his discretion, and thus still the cries which would otherwise distract or shock his neighbours or the class before whom he is operating.

At the first sight Clause 5 appears to spare domestic animals, but what is the real effect ? Special restrictions are indeed placed in the case of horses, asses, and mules. No person without a certificate complying with the terms of this section can operate upon them at all, with or without anæsthetics. But dogs and cats, most highly sensitive to pain, are handed over with no *special* restrictions to the simple licensee. They are naturally the favoured victims in private laboratories.

By Clause 21, even the enforcement of the provisions of the Act is left discretionary. No doubt public opinion would demand that the assent to prosecute should be given by the Secretary of State, if good cause were shown to believe that the Act had been materially infringed. Still consent may be legally refused.—*Abridged and digested from " Commentary on the Cruelty to Animals Act*, 1876 " (London, 1883).

ACT, The.   Cobbe.

FRANCES POWER COBBE, Authoress, Hengwrt, Dolgelly. (A.V.)

" Mr. Cartwright said, that ' the provisions of the Act made it impossible to operate except in a public place.'

" The ' provisions of the Act ' do no such thing. There is nothing concerning public places in them. All the laboratories in the kingdom are sufficiently private for anything anybody could reasonably desire to do in them ; and in several cases private residences have been licensed for vivisection, *e.g.* one in Queen Anne Street, London, and another at 35, Park Road South, Birkenhead."—*Comments on the Debate in the House of Commons,* April 4th, 1883, etc., by Frances Power Cobbe (London, 1883), p. 11.

—— The same.   Cobbe.

FRANCES POWER COBBE, Authoress, Hengwrt, Dolgelly. (A.V.)

" The most important of Mr. Cartwright's distinct misstatements is that concerning the Cat and Dog Clause in the Vivisection Act. According to the verbatim report, taken for the *Zoophilist,* Mr. Cartwright said—

" ' No cat, dog, horse, ass, or mule can be operated upon without a specific certificate for the purpose, and then only on the approval of the Home Secretary.''

" According to the *Times* report, he said to the same purpose :—

" ' It was further provided that no cat, dog, horse, mule, or ass, could be operated upon.'

" I cannot but wonder whether any statement as distinctly false as this, respecting an existing law under immediate debate, was ever imposed upon Parliament. When we reflect that Sir William Harcourt sat close by Mr. Cartwright during this speech, and witnessed this misleading of the House, and yet neither then, nor when he himself rose to speak on the same side, attempted to correct it—our confidence in the candour of the administrator of the law, or else in his acquaintance with the law which he administers, must, one or other, be rudely shaken.

" Here is what the Act really says, Clause 5 :—

" ' Notwithstanding anything in this Act contained, an experiment calculated to give pain shall not be performed *without anæsthetics* on a dog or cat, except on such certificate being given as in this Act mentioned . . . . and an experiment calculated to give pain shall not be performed on any horse, ass, or mule except on such certificate being given.'

" The two words marked in italics were inserted into the original Bill (which had placed all the five animals under like special protection) under the pressure of the 2,000 doctors who memorialized Sir Richard Cross on the 10th July, 1876. So hastily was this done that the margin still bears the original note ' *Special restrictions on painful experiments on dogs, cats. etc.*'—although, by means of this insidious interpolation, all special restrictions on experiments on dogs and cats were removed. while they were still left on experiments on horses, asses, and mules. As *no* vertebrate animal can, under the Act. be vivisected at all without the use (real or pretended) of anæsthetics, unless under special certificate for such purpose, dogs and cats are left by this clause, as it now stands, precisely in the same position as snakes, rats, and toads." [Nevertheless it is now the practice of the inspectors to give certificate ' E ' for experimenting on dogs and cats, and link it with certificate ' A ' dispensing with anæsthetics, or ' B ' dispensing with the obligation to kill the animal before recovery from anæsthesia. —F. P. C.' "—*Comments on the Debate in the House of Commons,* April 4th, 1883, *etc.*, by Frances Power Cobbe (London, 1883), pp. 4–5.

ACT, The, Experiments under.   Berdoe.

EDWARD BERDOE, M.R.C.S., L.R.C.P.Ed., London.   (A.V.)

On the Kidneys.—" Most of those who have taken any interest in this controversy, will remember the terrible experiments of Professor Roy on the circulation of the kidney. Divested of technicalities, they consisted in cutting down through the loins of living dogs and dissecting out their kidneys, but without dividing the veins and arteries by which they were connected to the circulatory system. A kidney-shaped metal box was made to fit the kidneys, which were placed in the box and surrounded with warm oil, the organs being then connected with delicate apparatus and recording instruments. Dr. Roy's invention has been a prolific source of suffering to countless animals. It has been taken up by Drs. Phillips and Bradford, who in August, 1887, in the pages of the *Journal of Physiology*, described their experiments with ' Roy's renal plethysmograph ' ' on the circulation and secretion of the kidney at the laboratory of University College, London.' Now it is well known that the kidney is one of the most delicate and sensitive organs in the body. There is a malady known as stone in the kidney, the suffering from which is often most excruciating. I have known patients writhe in agony on the floor of their bedroom when in paroxysms of pain from this cause, which is described in medical works as ' intense ; ' yet it can be nothing in comparison with the sufferings inflicted on these poor animals in Roy's experiments, although some amount of anæsthesia was induced."—*Twelve Years' Trial of the Vivisection Act, etc.*, by M.R.C.S. (London, 1889), pp. 7–8.

On the Brain.—" Again, everybody has heard of Ferrier's experiments upon the brains of living monkeys, but everybody does not know that these experiments are being daily repeated in London. I have before me *The Philosophical Transactions of the Royal Society of London*, vol. 179 (1888), B. pp. 303–327, recording an Investigation into the Functions of the Occipital and Temporal Lobes of the Monkey's Brain, by Sanger Brown, M.D., and E. A. Schäfer, F.R.S., Jodrell Professor of Physiology in University College, London. Here we have the old story of boring large holes into the skulls of monkeys, and burning out with a cautery, heated by the galvanic battery, large portions of their brains. When the operation had been successfully performed upon one side of the poor animal's head, ' a week after the first,' says the report, ' the same lesion [hurt or injury] was established on the other side of the brain.' The object of these dreadful injuries [made while the animal was

under the influence of chloroform] was to ascertain what effect
the destruction of different portions of the brain would have
upon the taste, sight, or hearing of the creature. Five weeks
after the second operation a third was performed, when mortification of the leg set in, 'and it was judged advisable to kill the
animal.' "—*Twelve Years' Trial of the Vivisection Act, etc.* By
" M.R.C.S." (London, 1889), pp. 9–10.

On the Sciatic Nerve.—" In February, 1887, Dr. Pye
Smith tells, in the *Journal of Physiology*, how, for six years, he ·
had been engaged in cutting down upon the sympathetic nerves
in the necks of cats and rabbits. In one rabbit, he says, the
sciatic nerve was cut down upon and tied, then it was subjected
to electrical stimulation, then the two vagi nerves were treated
in the same manner. Next, the left sympathetic (the right had
been operated upon previously) was similarly treated, and at
last the animal's chest was opened, and the heart examined.
After all these things had been done the animal was killed.
This long investigation was not carried on under the influence
of chloroform—that would have interfered with the result; the
very imperfect and unsatisfactory chloral had to be used.
Chloral is an uncertain drug under any circumstances, and
though a sleep producer it is not a true anæsthetic."—*Twelve
Years' Trial of the Vivisection Act, etc.* By "M.R.C.S." (London,
1889), pp. 11–12.

Freezing to Death.—" We may invite your attention to the
lecture delivered at the Royal Institution on Friday, May 29th,
1885, by Mr. J. J. Coleman, ' On the Mechanical Production of
Cold.' This gentleman related what he called the ' interesting experiments ' of Dr. McKendrick in freezing frogs and
rabbits to death. Placed in a cold chamber of 100° *below zero*,
in an hour's time, he says, the animal dies! When the story
was told, the distinguished and highly scientific audience
laughed derisively at the assurance of the lecturer that ' the
interesting experiment had nothing to do with vivisection.'
Yet, probably, there was not a scientific Englishman in the
room who would not have been ready at a moment's notice
to assure any of our sympathisers that ' it is only on the Continent that they do such dreadfully cruel things, you know !' "
—*Twelve Years' Trial of the Vivisection Act, etc.* By " M.R.C.S."
(London, 1889), p. 15.

On Consumption—with Public Money.—" In ' The Supplement to the Sixteenth Annual Report of the Local Government Board' we find Dr. Klein and Mr. A. Lingard actually
fed fowls upon the putrid lungs of human beings, to see if it
were possible thus to communicate to them the consumption of

which the human patients died. This loathsome series of experiments was carried out at the public expense, there being, as Mr. John Simon explained to the Royal Commission in 1875, an annual grant of £2.000, one-half of which was applied to this class of experiments."—*Twelve Years' Trial of the Vivisection Act, etc.*, by " M.R.C.S." (London, 1889), p. 16.

ACT, The, Experiments under   Lloyd Morgan.

C. LLOYD MORGAN, Principal at University College, Bristol. (V.)

" I will now briefly describe the nature of my experiments : (1) Condensing a sunbeam on various parts of the scorpion's body. . . . (2) Heating in a glass bottle, as this admits of most careful watching. I have killed some twenty or thirty individuals in this way. . . . (3) Surrounding with fire or red-hot embers. . . . (4) Placing in burning alcohol . . . (5) Placing in concentrated sulphuric acid. . . . The creature died in about ten minutes. . . . Burning phosphorus on the creature's body. I placed a small pellet of phosphorus near the root of the scorpion's tail, and lit the phosphorus with the touch of a heated wire. . . . (7) Drowing in water, alcohol, and ether. . . . (8) Placing in a bottle with a piece of cotton wool moistened with benzine. (9) Exposing to sudden light. (10) Treating with a series of electric shocks. General and exasperating causes of worry. I think it will be admitted," Mr. Morgan goes on to say, " that some of these experiments were sufficiently barbarous (the sixth is positively sickening) to induce any scorpions who had the slightest suicidal tendency to find relief in self-destruction. I have in all cases repeated the experiments on several individuals."—*Nature*, Feb. 1st, 1883.

—— The same.   Kent.

A. F. STANLEY KENT, M.A., Physiological Laboratory, University Museum, Oxford. (V.)

EXCISION OF THE THYROID GLAND.—The following experiments, which look very much like a repetition of those made by Mr. Horsley a few years back, were reported to the Physiological Society at its meeting at Oxford, June 24th, 1893. There is no mention of anæsthetics having been used :—

CAT I.—Both Thyroids excised. Three weeks after operation there was a difficulty in swallowing, with a tendency to vomit. Ten minims of extract given subcutaneously. At ninth week convulsions, which were subdued by injection of

eight minims of extract. Alive and well four months after operation. CAT II.—Both Thyroids excised. Died on third day. CAT IV.—Both Thyroids excised. On the fifteenth day distress. Ten minims of extract given. On sixteenth day thirty-five minims given in four doses. Its effect was very marked in reviving an apparently dead animal. Died on the seventeenth day. CAT V.—Both Thyroids excised. On fourth day convulsions. Ten minims of extract. On fifth day convulsions. Died. The extract did good, but could not save animal. Died on fifth day. CAT VI.—Both Thyroids excised. On sixteenth day very weak. Eight minims extract. No convulsions. Died. Pus in neck contains large bacillus and diplococcus. Temperature went up on day of death to 103.6. Leg ulcerated. Died on sixteenth day. CAT VII.—Treated with extract for ten days before operation. Both Thyroids excised. On fifth day very shaky. Sixteen minims extract. Feeding per rectum. Better sixth day. Fairly bright. Convulsions later. Seventh day eight minims extract. Died on eighth day.
— See " Proceedings of the Physiological Society," "Journal of Physiology," Vol. xv., p. 19 (1894).

ACT, The, Experiments under.   Bayliss and Bradford.

W. M. BAYLISS, B.A., B.Sc., and JOHN ROSE BRADFORD, M.D., B.Sc., Physiological Laboratory, University College, London. (V.)

SECTION AND STIMULATION OF NERVES OF THE LIMBS, ETC.— " Dogs of from fifteen to twenty pounds in weight were used. They were anæsthetised with chloroform, and morphia was then injected subcutaneously in doses of about half a grain, and after the operative procedure was completed, curare was injected into the external jugular vein. The vagi (nerves) were divided, tracheotomy performed, the carotid artery on one side prepared and connected with a mercurial manometer in the usual manner. . . . In the experiments requiring the exposure of the nerve roots. . . . it will suffice to say that the spinal cord was opened by removal of the neural arches, the nerve tied outside the dura mater and divided centrally to the ligature, so that a considerable length of the peripheral end was available for excitation. It is to be understood that in these experiments the peripheral ends of both anterior and posterior roots were excited together."—Journal of Physiology, vol. xvi., p. 13 (1894).

ACT, The, Experiments under.

Bradford and Dean.

JOHN ROSE BRADFORD, M.D., B.Sc., and HENRY PERCY DEAN, M.S., B.Sc., Physiological Laboratory, University College, London. (V.)

EXPLORATIONS INTO THE CHESTS OF TWENTY-NINE DOGS.— " In our experiments medium-sized dogs, weighing from 15lbs. to 20lbs., were generally used ; occasionally the dogs were somewhat larger and heavier. The animals were anæsthetised with chloroform, and then a dose of about a grain of acetate of morphia was given hypodermically. In this way, as is well known, a perfect anæsthesia is produced. The necessary operations were then carried out, and when completed the animal was curarised, as small a dose of curare as possible being used, and artificial respiration was carried on in the usual manner. . . . In many experiments curare was not used, *i.e.* in some of the experiments on the action of drugs, and in those on the influence of the respiratory move-ments on the pulmonary blood pressure. In all cases, however, artificial respiration was necessary, owing to the thorax having been opened to expose the pulmonary artery." (pp. 37-8).

" The pulmonary artery is reached as follows : The branch of the artery distributed to the lower lobe of the left lung was selected by us because this artery is sufficiently long for the necessary manipulations, and because the vessel can be reached comparatively easily from the back, and without any greater disturbance of the thoracic contents than opening one pleural cavity, throwing this lower lobe of the left lung out of action by the ligature of its main artery. In order to expose the artery here, two or occasionally three ribs require to be resected, the apex of the lower lobe of the lung is then seized, and the artery prepared in the usual manner. . . . If the artery is not readily seen, the bronchus can be seized with catch forceps, and dragged up to the level of the wound in the chest wall, when the artery will be readily detected just above the bronchus. The artery is ligatured as distally as possible, and the ligature cut long so as to leave a thread, by means of which the vessel can be pulled up to the level of the wound in the chest wall. A small clip is then placed on the vessel as centrally as possible, and the cannula tied in. . . . (p. 38.)

" In the experiments involving the spinal nerve roots, ... the nerves were exposed inside the spinal canal by the removal of the neural arches, and excited externally to the *dura mater* after ligature and division centrally to the point

excited. In this way, as pointed out previously, a comparatively long length of tough nerve is available for excitation,but
of course anterior and posterior roots are both excited together.
. . . (p. 39)

" As a general rule two or three nerves were exposed in
each experiment, as it is not advisable to expose a greater
length of the spinal cord. The upper dorsal nerves (a series
extending from the second to the seventh dorsal) were the
nerves most frequently excited. . . . (p. 39.)

" In these, as in all experiments on the vaso-motor system,
it is essential to work with the smallest effective dose of curare,
owing to the well-known paralysing action of the drug on the
vaso-motor apparatus." (p. 39.)—*Journal of Physiology*, vol.
xv. (1894.)

ACT, THE—Grounds of objection to. Bell.

ERNEST BELL, London. (A.V.)

Objection is raised to the Act on the following grounds :—

1. Because under it are licensed the very men whose deeds
and writings a few years ago raised so strong a feeling of
abhorrence in the public mind that the Royal Commission was
called for. One of the witnesses who candidly admitted that
he had " no regard at all " for the animals' sufferings has been
regularly licensed since 1884.

2. Because when a man is once licensed there is absolutely
no limit in duration or intensity to the suffering he may inflict.

3. Because the qualifications for obtaining a licence do not
depend at all on the applicant's moral character, but wholly on
his scientific training ; and the members of the scientific
societies and the professors who vouch for its competence are
themselves vivisectors or in favour of the practice, and thus
they practically recommend each other.

4. Because all the inspectors hitherto appointed have been
vivisectors or keen partizans, one of them having called our
movement " a mischievous and senseless agitation."

5. Because the Parliamentary Returns, as their wording
shows, are compiled, not from personal observation, but from
the statements furnished by the vivisectors themselves.
Accounts of horrible experiments published in scientific
journals thus never appear in the Returns, or only in such a
form that they cannot be recognised.

6. Because curare, though not recognised as an anæsthetic,
may still be used in conjunction with real anæsthetics. The
administration of chloroform, morphia, etc., is well known to

c

be difficult, and to need the most careful watching ; but when the animal is rendered perfectly motionless by curare there is no means of telling whether the other drug is having any effect or not, or whether the curare is itself sufficiently strong to exercise an anæsthetic effect.

7. Because no licensed person can be prosecuted under the Act without " the consent in writing of the Home Secretary." Previous to this Act the vivisector was liable to be prosecuted under Martin's Act, but now he is safe ; and thus the Vivisection Act, instead of protecting the animals, in reality protects the offender.

8. Because it is not based on any definite principle, and the parties chiefly concerned, viz. the animals, have been considered least. It is in reality a compromise made in the hope of satisfying two opposing parties. To please the humanitarians vivisection is prohibited under heavy penalties ; to pacify the physiologists it is again allowed by a system of licences and certificates ; and between the two the animals' interests have been left out and they are practically worse off than before.

ACUPRESSURE.   Tait.

PROF. LAWSON TAIT, F.R C.S., LL.D., late Professor of Gynæcology, Queen's College, Birmingham. (A.V.)

" The conclusions of the experiments were quoted far and wide, were translated into foreign languages ; and everything looked as if ' acupressure ' was to reform the art of surgery. But it did not : it speedily died out, and I think has been almost forgotten. The explanation of this lay in the simple fact that the closure of a dog's artery is altogether a different process from that seen in the human vessel ; and my experiments were not only needless, but they were absolutely misleading."—*Birmingham Daily Post*, Dec. 12th, 1881.

AIR AND RESPIRATION.   Macaulay.

JAMES MACAULAY, M.A., M.D., F.R.C.S.Ed., London.   (A.V.)

" No painful experiments on animals were required to prove that atmospheric air is necessary for the maintenance of life ; nor that atmospheric air, by continued breathing, becomes vitiated and unfit for respiration ; nor that it is diminished in volume by respiration : nor to show the relation of animal and vegetable life in regard to the condition of the atmosphere. All these discoveries belong to chemistry, and were ascertained and proved by facts and occurrences in common life, and observed in ordinary course of scientific investigation. The sad tragedy of the Black Hole at Calcutta, and the frequent calamities from 'choke damp' in mines, proved the effects of vitiated air, without the stupid demonstration of throwing dogs into the *grotte del cane*, far less of 'experiments' by physiologists. When the interpretation of these facts was given, by the discoveries of Priestley and Lavoisier, it was a triumph of chemical, not of physiological science, and entirely apart from vivisection."—*Vivisection : A Prize Essay* (London, 1881), p. 42.

ALCOHOL—Varying Action of, on Men and Animals. Berdoe.

EDWARD BERDOE, M.R.C.S., L.R.C.P.Ed., London. (A.V.)

"Alcohol is used in medicine as a cordial stimulant. Physiologists are much divided in opinion as to the way it acts upon man and animals. Dr. Zimmerburg, experimenting upon cats, said it *lowered the pulse rate*. Dr. Wood says that he thinks 'there must be some fallacy underlying' these experiments.

※   ※   ※   ※

"Dr. Ringer says :—'Observations on the influence of alcohol on the blood and organs have yielded contradictory results, the most recent and elaborate investigations of Parkes and Wollowicz clashing in most particulars with those of previous experimenters.' "—*Therapeutics*, p. 274, 5th ed.

"Dr. Ringer (himself a well-known experimenter) admits that 'as physiology fails to guide our steps amid these conflicting statements, we must rely solely on experience.'—*Therapeutics*, p. 277, 5th ed."—*The Futility of Experiments with Drugs on Animals*, by Edward Berdoe (London, 1889), pp. 8-9.

ALCOHOL. Various.

The Norwich experiments of Dr. Magnan in 1875, sworn at the prosecution, by Sir Wm. Fergusson, to be useless, were partly made with alcohol and partly with absinthe. In the *Revue des Deux Mondes*, for January, 1887, M. Haussonville, writing on *Le Combat contre le Vice*, tells us :—" L'alcool par lui même est un poison. M. le docteur Dujardin-Beaumetz a établi ce fait d'une façon irréfragable par une série d'expériences bien conduites *qui ont abouti à la mort de deux cent cinquante huit chiens* " (p. 132).

ALCOHOL—Experiments with, on Human Beings.   Ringer.

SYDNEY RINGER, M.D., M.R.C.S., Professor at University College, London.   (V.)

In Dr. Ringer's *Handbook of Therapeutics*, eighth edition, pp. 340-1 (as quoted in a letter in the *Standard*, November 19th, 1883, *à propos* of Ringer and Murrell's experiments on patients in hospitals), there are recorded other series of experiments conducted on human patients—not ending in death, indeed, but all, too probably, in utter demoralization. " Dr. Rickards and I," the author says, " gave to an habitual drunkard, making him dead drunk, 12 ounces of good brandy in a single dose. . . . . Drs. Parkes and Wollowicz gave to a healthy young man 12 ounces of brandy daily for three days." . . . " In a boy, aged 10, who had never in his life before taken alcohol in any form, I found, through a large number of observations, a . . . . reduction of temperature."

AMMONIUM, CHLORIDE OF (Sal Ammo-   Berdoe.
niac)—Contradictions of Experimenters.

EDWARD BERDOE, M.R.C.S., L.R.C.P.Ed., London.   (A.V.)

"Arnold found that 30 grains would kill a rabbit in ten minutes.

"Sundelin and Böcker (*Beitrage zur Heilkunde*, Bd. ii., p. 170) and other experimenters say that chloride of ammonium impoverishes the blood.

" Dr. Rabateau (*L'Union Médicale*, 1871, p. 330) injected the same drug into the veins of dogs with no apparent effect.

" Wood says (*Materia Medica*, p. 527) that ' although I have given the drug very largely and freely,' he has not found evidences of this action."—*The Futility of Experiments with Drugs on Animals*, by Edward Berdoe (London, 1889), p. 10.

AMYL, NITRITE OF.—*See* NITRITE OF AMYL.

ANÆSTHETICS AND CURARE—Why   Brunton.
these cannot be used together.

THOMAS LAUDER BRUNTON, M.D., D.Sc., Lecturer on Materia Medica, St. Bartholomew's Hospital, London.   (V.)

" Is there anything to prevent your giving both drugs, or giving them mixed together, so as to stop the pain by the chloroform and the nervous movement by wourali [curare]?

" Yes, there is, and it is this : in very many of those experiments you want to ascertain what is termed the reflex action ; that is to say, that an impression is made upon a nerve, and goes up to the cord, and is transmitted down. Now, chloroform acts upon the reflex centres, and abolishes their influence completely ; so that if you give the wourali, which paralyses the ends of the motor nerves, and give the chloroform, which paralyses the reflex centres, you deprive yourself of the possibility, in many instances, of making satisfactory experiments.

" But are there not many instances in which you give wourali simply for the purpose of getting the animal perfectly quiet ?

" Yes, those instances which I gave.

" But if it is done for the purpose of getting the animal perfectly quiet, could not chloroform be given also ?

" No, for that very reason ; if you were to give chloroform, the experiment would be at an end ; you would have abolished the action of the reflex centres, and thus you might as well not do the experiment at all."—*Evid. Roy. Com.* (London, 1876). Q. 5,743-5,745.*

ANÆSTHETICS—Antiseptics not Anæsthetics.   J. H. Clarke.

JOHN H. CLARKE, M.D., Physician to the Homœopathic Hospital, London. (A.V.)

" That it should be necessary to distinguish two things which have nothing in common except a similarity in the sound of the name, is due to the fact that vivisectors have persistently traded on public ignorance, and endeavoured, not without some success, to confuse the two in the public mind. 'The animals suffered little or no pain, since antiseptic precautions were observed,' is the kind of phrase generally met with.

" *Antiseptics* means a system of treating wounds so as to exclude from them the germs of putrefaction. It is derived from the Greek words ἀντι, against, and σηψις, putrefaction.

" *Anæsthetics* are agents which deprive sentient creatures of sensation. The term is derived from ἀν, a privative particle, and αἰσθησις, feeling.

" *Antiseptics* do nothing whatever to deaden feeling. An operation under antiseptic precautions is just as painful as

---

* Dr. Brunton afterwards sought unsuccessfully to modify the effect of this evidence. The contradictions he gave are exposed in "The Modern Rack" (London, 1889) pp., 142, 143.

without them. Before the antiseptic theory was discredited as
it now is, wounds treated antiseptically during and after operation were supposed to heal more rapidly than others, and this
afforded the only crumb of excuse for those who have confused
the two terms ; but even this crumb of excuse exists no longer,
since the theory and practice have been abandoned in ordinary
surgery."—J. H. C.

ANÆSTHETICS.   Brunton.

THOMAS LAUDER BRUNTON, M.D., D.Sc. Lecturer on Materia
    Medica at St. Bartholomew's, London.   (V.)

Dr. Lauder Brunton, speaking of a very long and painful
experiment on the secretion and circulation in the sub-
maxillary gland, states : " I must say that you cannot do the
whole experiment under chloroform, you cannot show it as you
would under wourali (curare)."—*Evid. Roy. Com.* (London,
1876).   Q. 5,811.

—— The same.   Burrows.

SIR GEORGE BURROWS, Bart., M.D. (the late), ex-President of
    the Royal College of Physicians.   (V.)

" There are a certain class of experiments which cannot be
performed under anæsthetics."—*Evid. Roy. Com.* (London,
1876).   Q. 162.

—— The same.   Rutherford

WILLIAM RUTHERFORD, M.D., Professor of the Institutes of
    Medicine, Edinburgh University.   (V.)
" Could not that [experiment on the dog's bile duct with
drugs] have been performed under anæsthetics ?
" It could not have been performed, so far as I know, under
any other agent but curare, the object being to keep the
animal perfectly still.   I do not think chloroform, opium, or
ether could have been administered."—*Evid. Roy. Com.* Q.
2,908 and 2,932.

—— The same.   Fergusson.

SIR WILLIAM FERGUSSON, Bart., F.R.S. (the late), Ser-
    geant Surgeon to the Queen.   (Born 1808 ; died 1877.)   (A.V.)

" I have very strong ideas with reference to these experiments performed under anæsthesia, as being far less valuable.

I do not go in with that view, which is very prevalent, that these experiments may now be permitted because we have got anæsthesia to prevent the pain. The experiment is not of the smallest value during its performance. You cannot make a perfect experiment on the animal until it is in its normal condition."—*Evid. Roy. Com.* (London, 1876). Q. 1,077.

ANÆSTHETICS.   Foster.

MICHAEL FOSTER, M.D., F.R.S., Professor of Physiology in the University of Cambridge. (V.)

"This can only be shown in the higher animals, the cat or dog being best adapted for the purpose. The method adopted is this—the arches of one or two vertebræ are carefully sawn through, or cut through with the bone forceps, and the exposed roots very carefully freed from the connective tissue surrounding them. If the animals be strong, and have thoroughly recovered from the chloroform, and from the operation, irritation of the peripheral stump of the anterior root causes not only contraction in the muscles supplied by the nerve, but also movements in other parts of the body, indicative of pain or of sensations. On dividing the mixed trunk . . . the contractions . . . cease, but the general signs of pain or sensation still remain."— *Handbook of the Physiological Laboratory* (London, 1873), p. 403.

—— The same.   Gimson.

W. GIMSON GIMSON, M.D., M.R.C.S., Witham, Essex. (A.V.)

"If sensation is deadened or suspended by the use of anæsthetics, from the moment that the anæsthetic agent enters the system, the whole organization is removed from its normal condition; the data recorded during such a state cannot be deemed reliable, and must lead to fallacies in building up any theory. Nor is it fair or truthful to hold up anæsthetics as a gilded bait to lure on the unwary. To many the mention of chloroform, ether, *et alia*, conveys the idea of abolition of suffering—but ask the multitude, and evidence will at once be forthcoming that these blessings are not unmitigated boons, nay, that they are up to certain points extreme torture, and any one who has administered chloroform frequently to dogs must have seen this latter statement borne out with reference to them."—*Vivisections and Painful Experiments on Living Animals; their Unjustifiability* (London, 1879), p. 61.

ANÆSTHETICS. Hoggan.

GEORGE HOGGAN, M.B. (the late, born 1837 ; died 1891), a
witness before the Royal Commission of 1875. (R.)

" Now you have expressed in letters that have appeared in
the public press the opinion that anæsthetics on the whole have
been rather curses than benefits to animals ?—I have.   Will
you give me the grounds of that opinion, as briefly as you
can ?—Principally because, as I have explained in those letters
(which I have put in before the Commission), the public have
generally supposed that anæsthetics were used, and they did
not feel called upon to make any demonstration to save animals
from pain, and while the animals were suffering pain all the
time the public really thought that nothing of the kind was
going on, and consequently anæsthetics had served more to
lull the public than the animals.   Those are nearly my words.
And the reasons given why anæsthetics were not so much
used as they were supposed to be, were first, that anæsthetics
if given to animals in many cases bring about a fatal result
before the experiment can be concluded,—if given thoroughly,
that is to say ; in the second place, that anæsthetics cannot
very well be given unless a special assistant is there for the
purpose ; and that these two things together cause so much
annoyance to the experimenter that he does not take the
trouble of thoroughly anæsthetising the animals.   This leaves
out of sight that great class of experiments where anæsthetics
would interfere with the true result of the experiment ; and
these are very numerous."—*Evid. Roy. Com.* (London, 1876).
Q. 4,107–8.

—— The same. Hoggan.

GEORGE HOGGAN, M.B. (the late, born 1837 ; died 1891), a
witness before the Royal Commission of 1875. (R.)

" The incalculable advantages which mankind has derived
from chloroform as a means of destroying the sense of pain
have remained a dead letter as regards the lower animals, in
consequence of the very unsatisfactory state of our knowledge
of the line which separates insensibility from death, especially
in some of those classes of animals which are most generally
employed as the subjects of physiological experimentation.
Many of these die apparently before they can become insensible through chloroform, some of them, indeed, as soon as
it has been administered.   The practical consequence of this
uncertainty is, that complete and conscientious anæsthesia is

seldom even attempted, the animal getting at most a slight whiff of chloroform, by way of satisfying the conscience of the operator, or of enabling him to make statements of a humane character."—*Letter in " The Spectator,"* May 29th, 1875.

ANÆSTHETICS.   Hoggan.

GEORGE HOGGAN, M.B. (the late, born 1837 ; died 1891), a witness before the Royal Commission of 1875. (R.)

" We fearlessly affirm that none of the following classes of experiments (each including innumerable operations, many of which involve extreme torture) can be performed under complete and genuine anæsthesia :—

" 1.   Those experiments which are concerned with the reflex action from the sensory nerves.

" 2.   Those which are connected with the glandular secretions, the liver, etc.

" 3.   Those on the digestion.

" 4.   Those on the heart and circulation.

" 5.   Toxicological experiments (poisons).

" 6.   All pathological experiments (consisting in the artificial induction of disease)."—*" Anæsthetics and Vivisection : " The Zoophilist*, May, 1885.

—— The same.   Klein.

EMMANUEL KLEIN, M.D., F.R.S., Lecturer on Anatomy and Physiology, St. Bartholomew's Medical School, London. (V.)

" I suppose with rabbits you would not use chloroform ?—I use chloral hydrate ; but, as a general rule, for my scientific investigations, I do not use chloroform, or any other anæsthetic, except for convenience sake, in dogs and cats, and for no other animals as a general rule.   There may be exceptions, perhaps ; but, as a general rule, I think I am safe in saying I do not use it.   You gave it as your opinion, that your views on the subject, although not shared by the British public generally, were the views of the British physiologists ?—I would not say that distinctly, but I know a few of them, and I think that is the view held by them."—*Evid. Roy. Com.* (London, 1876). Q. 3,605–6.

—— The same.   McDonnell.

ROBERT McDONNELL, M.D., F.R.S. (the late), Dublin. (V.)

" In this particular class of cases the experiments are on sensation [nerves] ; the pain could not be avoided, therefore

in that particular class of cases. Are there any of those which
you have practised yourself in which there has been prolonged
pain ?—No, not prolonged pain, but unavoidable pain. I have
repeated at the time that they were quite new and *sub judice*,
the researches of Dr. Brown-Séquard upon the spinal cord of
animals. In those cases I believe it is unavoidable to have
suffering."—*Evid. Roy. Com.* (London, 1876). Q. 4,487–8.

ANÆSTHETICS. Watson.

SIR THOMAS WATSON, Bart., M.D. (the late) Past President of the
Royal College of Physicians (born 1792, died 1882). (V.)

" *Lord Winmarleigh:* We may presume that in those experiments [Sir C. Bell's on the nerves] the use of anæsthetics
is quite useless, that it would be of no effect ?—They would
defeat the object of the experiment. (Q. 49.)
" *Sir John Karslake:* I wished to ask you whether any other
cases suggest themselves to you than those which you have
last described in which the use of anæsthetics would frustate
the object of the experiment ? . . . I should think that the
use of anæsthetics might vitiate the results of any trials of
poisons upon animals."—*Evid. Roy. Com.* (London, 1876). Q.
54–5.

—— The same. Schafer.

EDWARD ALBERT SCHAFER, M.R.C.S., F.R.S., Jodrell Professor of Physiology, University College, London. (V.)

"Then may I take it there are a great number of experiments which, supposing a frog to be a sensitive animal, must
cause a vast deal of pain, which are not done under
chloroform ?—There is no doubt of it. And there is no
precaution taken to diminish pain, if it suffers pain ?—I think
I may say no special precaution."—*Evid. Roy. Com.* (London,
1878.) Q. 3,801–2.

—— The same—Experiments on the nerves cannot be done under anæsthetics.—*See* NERVES.

—— Nitrous oxide. Gimson.

W. GIMSON GIMSON, M.D., M.R.C.S., Witham, Essex. (A.V.)

" The modern history of anæsthetics dates back to the end
of the last century, when the discoveries of Priestley,
Black, and Cavendish, created a new era in the chemical

world, and gave rise to a new branch of therapeutics,
called *pneumatic medicine*, whose votaries hoped to cure
diseases, and especially consumption, by the inhalations of
various kinds of gases. In following out this theory, Humphry, afterwards Sir Humphry Davy, was, about 1800, led
to the conclusion that 'nitrous oxide (laughing gas)
appeared capable of destroying physical pain, so it might
probably be used with advantage during surgical operations.
This conclusion was arrived at by experiments upon himself
and not upon animals. Not until the year 1844 was the use of
this anæsthetic established, when a dentist, Horace Wells,
acting upon Davy's suggestion, inhaled the nitrous oxide
himself before one of his teeth was extracted, with the effect
of producing a complete unconsciousness of pain ; he also
administered it to several patients with the same beneficial
results."—*Vivisections and Painful Experiments on Living
Animals* (London, 1879), pp. 126-7.

ANÆSTHETICS. Pritchard.

WILLIAM PRITCHARD, M.R.C.V.S., (the late), Prof. Royal
Veterinary College. (A.V.)

" Does your experience extend to dogs ?—Yes. What is your
opinion about the sort of questions which I have put to you
when applied, not to horses, but to dogs ?—With regard to dogs,
I should never think of applying chloroform at all ; I should
think it very unsafe to do so. The dog has an intermittent
pulsation ; the heart's action is intermittent.

" *Lord Winmarleigh :* Invariably ?—Invariably. They appear
for some time not to be under the influence of it at all, and then
suddenly they come under the influence of it, and we find it
impossible to bring them round. Does any cruelty attach to
the death under those circumstances ?—I should say not ; it is
an awkward thing for the operator and for the owner.

" *Mr. Forster :* With regard to cats, what should you say as
to the use of chloroform ?—I have never administered it to
cats ; I do not think there would be the same risk.

" *Chairman :* Supposing you had a painful operation to
perform on a cat, you would use anæsthetics ?—I think so.

❊   ❊   ❊   ❊   ❊

" *Chairman :* Do I rightly understand you to say that the
circulation of the dog being intermittent, there is much more
danger that the animal would never revive than there would be
in the human being ?—Quite so."—*Evid. Roy. Com.* (London,
1876). Q. 796-803.

ANÆSTHETICS.   Rolleston.

GEORGE ROLLESTON (the late), M.D. Oxon., 1857, F.R.C.P.,
F.R.S., Linacre Prof. of Anatomy at Oxford (born 1829 ; died
1890). (V.)

" It is not so easy a thing to know when you have an animal
thoroughly anæsthetised ; and what is more, some animals
recover with much greater rapidity than others of the same
species from the same doses of anæsthetics." . . . "The
whole question of anæsthetising animals has an element of
uncertainty about it."—*Evid. Roy. Com.* (London, 1876). Q.
1,349-50.

—— The same.   Rutherford.

WILLIAM RUTHERFORD, M.D. Edin., M.R.C.S. Eng., Professor of the Institutes of Medicine, University of Edinburgh. (V.)

" What is the rule by which you guide yourself in determining
whether animals shall be rendered insensible to pain or not ?—
When the mode of rendering them insensible to pain would
interfere with the due result being obtained from the experiment, we do not so render them. Is that any large proportion
of the experiments ?—I should say a considerable proportion.
Would it be more than half the experiments ?—I should have
a difficulty in saying how many, but I should think about
half the experiments that I have done."—*Evid. Roy. Com.*
(London, 1876). Q. 2,841-3.

—— The same.   Walker.

ARTHUR DE NOÉ WALKER, M.R.C.S., London, a Witness
before the Royal Commission, 1875. (A.V.)

" When an experimenter says, for example, as is said in
a very recent publication, that ' before and throughout these
experiments anæsthetics were used,' it is perfectly true : but if
by that you choose to understand that while the animal lived
and was experimented on he was throughout insensible, it is
the greatest delusion that ever was."—*Evid. Roy. Com.*
(London, 1876). Q. 1810.

[As, for instance, in Mr. Horsley's experiments for the
Hydrophobia Committee, in a footnote of his report (Appendix
A of Report) he says :—"All the experiments performed in
this inquiry were thus " (alluding to the giving of chloroform)
" made painless." Here Mr. Horsley should have said
operations, not *experiments* ; for while the animal had chloroform

for the operative portion of the experiment, it suffered the disease of rabies, unrelieved, of course, by any anæsthetics.— *S. Harris*, M.R.C.S.]

ANEURISM—Hunter and tying for. Fergusson.

SIR WILLIAM FERGUSSON, F.R.S. (the late), Sergeant Surgeon to the Queen (born 1808; died 1877). (A.V.)

"John Hunter, who was one of our greatest physiologists, and allowed to be one of our greatest surgeons also, and may be said to this day to stand at the head of what is called scientific surgery in this country, is specially celebrated for an operation which he devised on the arteries. That operation for sixty or eighty years stood as one of the most brilliant in surgery : and in so far as I have been able to make out (and I have inquired into the subject), Hunter's first experiment, if it might so be called, was done on the human subject, and it was long after he had repeated his operation on the human subject, and others had repeated it, that the fashion of tying arteries on the lower animals originated or was developed. That fashion was quite justifiable at the time; it is no longer now justifiable ; but in regard to the surgical aspect of the case, the experiment might have been left entirely untouched, for Hunter had already experimented and developed the fact on the human subject. Then in short in this particular case the experiments that were tried on living animals did not establish the fact; they were only useful, if at all, for illustrating it *a posteriori ?*—Quite so."—*Evid. Roy. Com.* (London, 1876). Q. 1,024-5.

—— The same—Hunter and tying for. Gimson

W. GIMSON GIMSON, M.D., M.R.C.S., Witham, Essex. (A.V.)

"An aneurism may be described as a tumour filled with blood, from the rupture, wound, ulceration, or simple dilatation of an artery : having a tendency to increase, and to ultimately cause death by hæmorrhage. Cases have been found in which nature has proved sufficiently powerful to effect a cure, but these form the exception. The great physiologist Haller had asserted that he could imitate in animals the formation of an aneurism, and that he could readily produce one by separating the fibrous coat from the inner coat of an artery. John Hunter denied that this could be done; he laid bare the carotid artery (of a dog), afterwards 'skinned it with a knife even to transparency,' but no dilatation of the vessel took place : on the contrary, the vessel was rendered stronger, as Hunter declared it would be, in consequence of the adhesive inflammation taking place. Haller, in his experiments, left the denuded vessel to remain isolated and separated from the adjoining soft parts: Hunter allowed the artery and the surrounding cellular tissue to unite, and hence the difference in the results obtained by these experimenters. The earliest case of which the particulars are recorded, amounting to a satisfactory proof, of the application of the ligature for the cure of an aneurism, is the example, related by M. Severinus, of a false aneurism of the thigh, caused by a musket-ball wound. In this instance, Severinus tied the femoral artery above and below the aperture in it, and not only was the patient's life saved, but the use of the limb was also preserved. The next authentic case of the ligature of the femoral artery is that reported by Saviard, where Bottentuit, in 1668, tied this artery on account of a false aneurism, the result of a sword wound, at the inner and upper part of the thigh. A ligature was placed above, and another below the wound in the vessel: the patient recovered and enjoyed good health. . . . The application of the ligature for the cure of aneurism, viz. the cutting down upon the tumour, turning out the contents, and securing both ends of the vessel, yielded most unsatisfactory results; and it was not until John Hunter, in 1785, practised an operation the result of careful reasoning, that any real advance was made. Hunter believed that aneurismal arteries were usually diseased, and therefore he applied his ligature at a distance from the swelling, and did not open the tumour at all; his principles of adhesion and absorption, powers which he had learned to recognise, were the physiological resources on which he relied for the gradual disappearance of the tumour, so as to render any opening of it unnecessary."—*Vivisections and Painful Experiments on Living Animals: their Unjustifiability* (London, 1879), pp. 15–17.

ANEURISM—Hunter and tying for.   Macilwain.

GEORGE MACILWAIN, F.R.C.S. (the late), a Witness before the Royal Commission, 1875 (born, 1797 ; died, 1882). (A.V.)

" I see it is stated that John Hunter made experiments on animals. Undoubtedly he did.

But . . . there was not one single thing that he discovered or did, or a single conclusion that he drew from experiments on animals, that might not be much more clearly proved by the ordinary practice of surgeons. . . . . An aneurism is a giving way of the internal coat of an artery; . . . . but there is an aneurism, which is the ordinary case, which consists in the giving way of the internal coat of the vessel. The blood becomes then propelled against the yielding coat; the blood forms a pulsating tumour, and that is what we call an aneurism. Up to that time I must tell you that the operation on that disease was a very formidable operation, and too frequently fatal. It consisted in opening the sac and tying the artery on both sides of it. This was found to be a very bad operation, frequently attended with fatal consequences. I need not detain you with telling you the process. Now Mr. Hunter said that the cause of that was that the artery was tied in a spot where it was diseased, and that if he tied the artery in a sound part, he would most likely find that the thing would do very well. He accordingly did so, and the operation proved successful; and that has been certainly a very desirable and excellent improvement in the practice of surgery. But there was not a single thing with regard to it that he could have discovered in a living animal. Now the thing which has probably caused some unthinking persons to infer that is this. There was a great contest at the time. They said that Mr. Hunter was wrong, and that the arteries were generally diseased. Then Mr. Hunter made an experiment on an animal; that is to say, he tried to make an aneurism. He bared an artery, and he dissected off the coats of the artery, only leaving the internal coat, so as to make it as weak as he could, and then he bound up the wound; but after a time he killed the animal, opened the wound, and found that everything had healed, just as if nothing had been the matter. In fact, he could not make an aneurism; and as animals do not have aneurisms, but only the human subject, it is quite clear that there is not a shadow of shade of evidence that his discovery was the result of experiments on animals."—*Evid. Roy. Com.* Q. 1,845-6 (p. 96, col. 2; p. 97, col. 1).

ANEURISM—Hunter and tying for. Tait.

LAWSON TAIT, F.R.C.S., late Professor of Gynæcology, Queen's College, Birmingham. (A.V.)

"This illustration [of the value of vivisection] has been so completely and so often destroyed, that it is absolutely unnecessary to allude to it further than to explain that Hunter modified Anel's operation merely because he found the artery near to the seat of disease would not hold the ligature, and the patients bled to death. As the arteries of animals never suffer from the disease in question, experiments upon them could not have helped Hunter in any way whatever. Sir James Paget, who has lately appeared as an ardent advocate for vivisection, and, therefore, may be appealed to by me as a witness not biassed to my view, has recorded his opinion in the Hunterian oration given at the College of Surgeons in 1877, that Hunter's improvement in the treatment of aneurism ' was not the result of any laborious physiological induction ; it was mainly derived from facts very cautiously observed in the wards and deadhouse.' In this opinion Sir James Paget is undoubtedly correct."—*The Uselessness of Vivisection*, New Ed. (London, 1883), p. 22. " Hunter tried his best to induce aneurism on the lower animals and failed."—*The same Book*, p. 34.

ANGINA PECTORIS.—*See* NITRITE OF AMYL.

ANIMAL EXTRACTS, Treatment with. "Lancet."
" THE LANCET," Medical Newspaper, London. (P.V.)

" We feel, when such a competent physician as M. Constantin Paul goes so far as to treat mental disease by injections of ' cerebin ' and chronic renal disease by ' nephrine ' (an emulsion of the kidneys), that the limits of rational medicine are being overstepped. There are few affections like myxœdema, where the absence of an organ concerned in nutrition is the constant pathological feature ; and few, therefore, in which the principle of treatment illustrated by these attempts is likely to be of real practical value."—" *The Lancet*," Feb. 4th, 1893, p. 256.

ANIMALS' RIGHTS.—EARLY TESTI- MONIES. Hildrop.
JOHN HILDROP, M.A., Rector of Wath, near Ripon, Yorks. (A.V.)

Some serious writers upon this subject tell you that their (animals') existence was given them upon this very condition, that it should be temporary and short, that after they had flutter'd, or crept, or swam, or walk'd about their respective elements for a little season, they should be swept away by the hand of violence, or the course of nature, into an entire extinction of being, to make room for their successors in the same circle of vanity and corruption. But, pray, who told them so ? Where did they learn this philosophy ? Does either reason or revelation give the least countenance to such a bold assertion ?

So far from it, that it seems a direct contradiction to both."—
"*Free Thoughts upon the Brute Creation,*" *by John Hildrop, M.A.*
(*London,* 1742).

ANIMALS' RIGHTS.   Primatt.

REV. HUMPHREY PRIMATT, D.D., London.   (A.V.)

"However men may differ as to speculative points of religion,
justice is as a rule of universal extent and invariable obligation.
We acknowledge this important truth in all matters in which
Man is concerned, but then we limit it to our own species
only." (p. 1). . . . He applies to the animal question the
precept of *doing to others as we would be done unto,* and continues, "If, in *brutal* shape, *we* had been endued with the same
degree of reason and reflection which we now enjoy ; and other
beings, in *human* shape, should take upon them to torment,
abuse, and barbarously ill-treat us, because we were not made
in their shape ; the injustice and cruelty of their behaviour to
us would be self evident ; and we should naturally infer that,
whether we walk upon two legs or four ; whether our heads
are prone or erect ; whether we are naked or covered with
hair ; whether we have tails or no tails, horns or no horns,
long ears or round ears ; or, whether we bray like an ass, speak
like a man, whistle like a bird, or are mute as a fish ; Nature
never intended these distinctions as foundatious for right of
tyranny and oppression." (pp. 17-18).—"*A dissertation on the
Duty of Mercy and Sin of Cruelty to Brute Animals,*" *by
Humphrey Primatt* (*London,* 1776).

—— The same.   Bentham.

JEREMY BENTHAM, Author, London (born 1748, died 1832).
(A.V.)

"If the being killed were all, there is very good reason why
we should be suffered to kill such animals as molest us we
should be the worse for their living, and they are never the
worse of being dead.   But is there any reason why we should
be suffered to torment them ? Not any that I can see. Are
there any why we should *not* be suffered to torment them ?
Yes, several. The day has been, I grieve to say in many
places it is not yet past, in which the greater part of the
species, under the denomination of *slaves,* have been treated by
the law exactly upon the same footing as, in England, for
example, the inferior races of animals are still. The day *may*
come when the rest of the animal creation may acquire those
rights which never could have been withholden from them but

D

by the hand of tyranny. The French have already discovered that the blackness of the skin is no reason why a human being should be abandoned without redress to the caprice of a tormentor. It may come one day to be recognised that the number of the legs, the villosity of the skin, or the termination of the *os sacrum*, are reasons equally insufficient for abandoning a sensitive being to the same fate. What else is it should trace the insuperable line ? Is it the faculty of reason, or, perhaps, the faculty of discourse ? But a full-grown horse or dog is, beyond comparison, a more rational, as well as more conversable animal than an infant of a day, a week, or even a month old. But the question is not Can they *reason* ? nor Can they *talk* ? but, Can they *suffer* ? "—"*Introduction to the Principles of Morals and Legislation*," *by Jeremy Bentham* (London, 1789), p. 308, note.

ANIMALS' RIGHTS.   Young.

THOMAS YOUNG, Fellow of Trinity College, Cambridge. (A.V.)

" Animals are endued with a capability of perceiving pleasure and pain ; and from the abundant provision which we perceive in the world for the gratification of their several senses, we must conclude that the Creator wills the happiness of these his creatures, and consequently that humanity towards them is agreeable to him, and cruelty the contrary. This, I take it, is the foundation of the rights of animals, as far as they can be traced independently of scripture ; and is, even by itself, decisive on the subject, being the same sort of argument as that on which moralists found the Rights of Mankind, as deduced from the Light of Nature."—"*An Essay on Humanity to Animals*," *by Thomas Young* (London, 1798), p. 8.

—— The same.   Gompertz.

LEWIS GOMPERTZ, Secretary Society for the Prevention of Cruelty, 1826-32. (Died 1861). (A.V.)

" It is to be lamented that even philosophers frequently forget themselves on this subject, and relate, with the greatest indifference, the numerous barbarous and merciless experiments they have performed on the suffering and innocent brutes, even on those who show affection for them ; and then coldly make their observations and calculations on .every different form in which the agony produced by them manifests itself. But this they do for the advancement of science ! and expect much praise for their meritorious exertions ; forgetting that science should be subservient to the welfare of man and other animals, and ought not to be pursued merely through emulation, nor even for the sensual gratification the mind derives from them, at the expense of justice, the destruction of the happiness of others, and the production of their misery."— "*Moral Inquiries on the Situation of Man and the Brutes*" (London, 1824), pp. 8, 9.

ANIMALS' RIGHTS. Youatt.

WILLIAM YOUATT, Professor in the Royal Veterinary College (Died 1847). (A.V.)

" The claims of humanity, however they may be neglected or outraged in a variety of respects, are recognized by every ethical writer. They are truly founded on reason and on scripture, and in fact are indelibly engraven on the human heart. . . . Nevertheless, the claims of the lower animals to humane treatment, or at least to exemption from abuse, are as good as any that man can urge upon man. Although less intelligent, and not immortal, they are susceptible of pain : but because they cannot remonstrate, nor associate with their fellows in defence of their rights, our best theologians and philosophers have not condescended to plead their cause, or even to make mention of them ; although, as just asserted, they have as much right to protection from ill-usage as the best of their masters have."—*The Obligation and Extent of Humanity to Brutes, &c.*," by *W. Youatt* (London, 1839), introduction.

—: The same. Harold Browne.

RIGHT REV. HAROLD BROWNE (the late), Bishop of Winchester (born 1811 ; died 1891.) (A.V.)

" There were two parties, for whose protection they were interested. He ventured to call them both his friends, and he believed those assembled would do so likewise. First, the brute creatures—many of them were amongst the warmest friends of mankind, our dumb, and, as people called them some·times, our ' poor relations ' ; although he did not see with freedom given to them they were poorer than mankind—indeed, they were oft times far richer. He maintained that we had no right to torture these creatures of God for the sake of any supposed benefit we might derive from doing so. He quite admitted that man was superior to the beast, but the part of him which was so valuable was not his bodily constitution but the immortal part of his being. Take that away and men were not much superior, that he could see, to animals. And it must be borne in mind that it was only for the good of their animal nature that they tortured these poor creatures. Further, they could inflict no greater suffering probably upon the brute creation than upon their bodies. He said probably, because some animals exhibited such superior instinct, combined with affection, as to make many doubt whether they were not gifted with higher natures than those usually attributed to them. Now, with man, mental suffering might be much greater than bodily suffering, and moral degradation was worse than all ; but with animals it was not so, and in inflicting upon them bodily suffering they were touching that part of their nature which was most susceptible to pain. He did not believe that for the mere sake of our bodily natures we were justified in this."—*Extract from a Speech at Southampton*, October 16th, 1878.

ANIMALS' RIGHTS. MORALS AND LOGIC.   Coleridge.

LORD COLERIDGE (The late), Lord Chief Justice of England. (Died 1894). (A.V.)

" As to man himself, it was not so long ago that medical men met with a passion of disavowal, what they regarded as an imputation, viz. the suggestion that experiments were tried on patients in hospitals. I assume the disavowal to be true ; but why, if all pursuit of knowledge is lawful, should the imputation be resented? The moment you come to distinguish between animals and man, you consent to limit the pursuit of knowledge by considerations not scientific but moral ; and it is bad logic and a mere *petitio principii* to assume (which is the very point at issue) that these considerations avail for man but do not for animals. I hope that morals may always be too much for logic ; it is permissible to express a fear that some day logic may be too much for morals."—*From " The ' Nineteenth Century ' Defenders of Vivisection,"* by Lord Coleridge (London, Victoria Street Society, 1893).

ANTHRAX AND INSURANCE.   Serle.

PHILIP SERLE, Esq., 22, Rue Matignon, Paris. (A.V.)

It has been stated in debate that offices engaged in the insurance of cattle in Paris had refused to issue policies where the animals had not been inoculated for anthrax by the Pasteurian method. Mr. Serle, by request, made inquiries as to this statement, and reported as follows :—" The ordinary Insurance Companies here do not insure live stock, but I got the addresses of some that do and went to them yesterday. They are *La Mutualité Générale, La Caisse des Propriétaires*, and the *Bétail.* They one and all assure me that such a thing as inoculation was never required by them, and the *Bétail* man was almost disposed to think that I had come to poke my fun at him."—*Letter from Mr. Serle, dated* September 8th, 1892.

ANTHRAX, Inoculation for.   Clarke.

JOHN H. CLARKE, M.D., Physician to the Homœopathic Hospital, London. (A.V.)

M. Pasteur's "results have been tested by other experiments in Hungary (by his own pupil and agent, the late M. Thuillier, watched by a Government Commission), in England (by Dr. Klein), in Germany (by Dr. Thuillier), and by others in France. The result of these several trials is, that all the observers agree that M. Pasteur's ' vaccinations' have a certain scientific interest, but from a practical point of view are not only value-less, but positively dangerous to man and beast. It is not denied that M. Pasteur's 'vaccines' protect against infection by inoculation, but it is proved that they are of no use against natural infection. It is also proved that they are of extremely uncertain strength, and of equally uncertain protective value, as against virulent inoculation. Also, they are far from being free from risk—a very considerable percentage of the animals dying from the 'vaccinations.' The Hungarian Commission recommended its Government to prohibit the use of M. Pasteur's 'vaccines'; and the German and English observers viewed them with no greater favour. Nearly all observers agree that M. Pasteur's theories regarding the etiology of the disease, and the cause of the attenuation of the virus, are completely erroneous."—*The Protective Value of Anthrax Vaccination* (London, 1886), pp. 3, 4.

—— The same.   Klein.

EMMANUEL KLEIN, M.D., F.R.S., Lecturer on Anatomy and Physiology, St. Bartholomew's Hospital, London. (V.)

" Regarding the protective power of inoculation, Dr. Klein asks the question : ' Is a cultivation in which in course of time the *bacillus anthracis,* at first forming a copious growth, degenerates, and in which no spores had been formed, and further which cultivation loses, as we know, its power to infect with virulent anthrax, animals when inoculated ;' that is to say, such a cultivation as M. Pasteur's *vaccins* profess to be :—' is such a cultivation, I say, perfectly ineffective too, in giving the animals some sort of immunity against further inoculation with virulent material?' The answer is simply—'Yes: it is perfectly ineffective.'"—*Supplement to the Twelfth Annual Report of the Local Government Board*, 1882-3, p. 208.

ANTHRAX.   Koch.

ROBERT KOCH, M.D., Professor of Hygiene, etc., Berlin. (V.)

"Experiment (*a*). Eight sheep which had been inoculated with protective *vaccin* after M. Pasteur's method, and one sheep that had not been so protected, were inoculated with active virus from a case of spontaneous charbon. In ten days one of the 'protected' sheep and the unprotected one were dead of charbon. (*b*) Twelve days after the control experiment, the seven surviving sheep and one which had not been inoculated were fed with potatoes in which spores were cultivated. Two of the seven, and the one uninoculated sheep died within two days. From this Dr. Koch concludes that natural infection is different from, and more fatal than, infection conveyed by inoculation ; and further, that the 'protective' inoculation with M. Pasteur's *vaccins* is of little avail against *natural* infection (p. 30)."—"*L'Inoculation Préventive du Charbon.*" *Reply to M. Pasteur* (Berlin, etc,, 1883).

—— The same.   Koch.

ROBERT KOCH, M.D., Professor of Hygiene, etc., Berlin. (V.)

"The preventive vaccination of Pasteur cannot be considered practically utilisable, on account of the insufficient preservation that it gives against natural infection, on account of the short duration of that preservation, and on account of the danger to which it subjects men and non-vaccinated animals."—"*L'Inoculation Preventive du Charbon.*" *Reply to M. Pasteur*, p. 35.

—— The same.   Colin.

M. COLIN, Professor at the French Veterinary School at Alfort. (V.)

"I was already acquainted with the results of the inoculations with the *virus charbonneux*, and they authorize my doubts as to the ultimate success of the hydrophobic inoculations. I had certainly succeeded in causing some individuals of certain species to become proof by these inoculations, but, at the same time, I had ascertained that this immunity did not extend to all cases, that its duration was limited and variable, and that, in fact, the inoculations might cause the malady to appear in a fatal way. This caused me to reflect, and I have never had any reason for changing the opinion I arrived at, namely, that they were going too fast, and were acting rashly in making a general prophylactic system out of these inoculations."— *Speech at the Academy of Medicine, Paris, Nov. 9th, 1886.*

ANTHRAX.—Fatality of Pasteurian   Lutaud. Inoculations for.

A. LUTAUD, M.D., Chief Editor of the *Journal of Medicine*, Paris. (V.)

" The statistical record of the mortality that has followed the treatment by anthrax vaccine is conclusive. Only a few among the thousands of facts available as evidence can be cited. In a farm in the environs of Laon, a flock attacked with anthrax was vaccinated as many as three times, at intervals of fifteen days without eradicating the disease. In a neighbouring farm horses suffering from no disease were vaccinated, and three perished as the result of the operation. The proprietor, M. Magnier, demanded the value of his horses, which was reimbursed to him. In the environs of Meaux, a veterinary surgeon having killed four cows with the famous vaccine, M. Pasteur paid for these animals, to cut short the abuse of the interested parties.

" Other examples, instanced by M. Paul Boullier, veterinary surgeon at Courville (Eure et Loir):—

" In 1882, M. Franchamp, agriculturist at Tremblay, canton of Châteauneuf (Eure et Loir), lost horses, cows, and sheep to the value of five thousand francs, the same having died in consequence of anthrax vaccination.

" In 1883, M. Fournier, veterinary surgeon at Angerville Loiret), vaccinated a flock of 400 sheep, and some days after the application of the No. 1 vaccine, ninety sheep succumbed from anthrax in the blood.

" Finally, in 1884, two of my clients and friends, M. Henri Thirouin, Mayor of Saint-Germain-le-Gaillard and M. Marcet Lebrun, agriculturist in the same district, were induced to vaccinate their sheep by one of my colleagues of Chartres, M. Ernest Boutet. They lost between them as many sheep as had died in the entire thirty districts in which I practice as a veterinary surgeon, and in which vaccination does not take place, and forty-five times more than the fifty other agriculturists have lost, who possess sheep at Saint-Germain-le-Gaillard."—From *Etudes sur la Rage*, by Dr. Lutaud (2nd edition, Paris, 1891), pp. 419–20.

ANTISEPTIC SURGERY—Lister's Spray.   Bantock.

GEORGE GRANVILLE BANTOCK, M.D., F.R.C.S.Ed., Senior
Surgeon Samaritan Free Hospital. (R.)

" In this country, at least, it is a very rare thing to see the
spray in use at all. For the most part it is to be seen put to
a purpose for which it was never intended by the inventor, *i.e.*
playing upon the ceiling or against a wall, or anywhere but on
the field of operation. This is at best a most illogical proceeding, and I am quite at a loss to understand the process of
reasoning—if there be any—which leads to such a practice. In
the Samaritan Free Hospital it has been discarded by all my
colleagues with one exception. I am making no assumption
when I say that this is due to the superior results which I
have obtained there since I reverted to a more rational and
more simple method. . . . I have frequently been asked,
' Would you open a knee-joint without an antiseptic?' My
answer has been, ' Yes, most certainly, if the opportunity
offered,' for I see no difference between the serous membrane
of the knee-joint and the abdominal cavity."—*Provincial Medical Journal*, Dec., 1889, pp. 721-2.

—— The same.   Clarke.

JOHN H. CLARKE, M.D., Physician to the Homœopathic Hospital,
London. (A.V.)

" Philanthropos . . . adduces the use of carbolic acid as
one of the fruits of vivisection, and consequently, also, the
whole system of antiseptic surgery. On this we briefly say:
(1) That Déclat used carbolic acid before Lister. (2) When we .
had the privilege of hearing Mr. Lister explain his antiseptic
theory, he informed us that he elaborated it principally by
means of experiments with *milk*. (3) Mr. Lister's assistant,
Mr. Watson Cheyne, has proved that the theory is all wrong,
that germs can live and flourish in the most 'aseptic' of
wounds, and sometimes delight themselves in solutions of carbolic acid ; and further, that abscesses which have never been
exposed to the air may be crowded with germs and living
organisms. (*Trans. Int. Med. Cong.*, 1881, i. 321.) (4) Not a
few lives have been lost by the indiscriminate use of carbolic
acid, and much harm has often been done by it both to patient
and surgeon, as was proved by the celebrated surgeon Mr.
Keith, at the International Congress. (*Trans.*, ii. 236.) "—
" *Physiological Cruelty*," a reply to " *Philanthropos*," London
1883.

ANTISEPTIC SURGERY—Lister's Spray.   Tait.

LAWSON TAIT, F.R.C.S., late Professor of Gynæcology, Queen's College, Birmingham. (A.V.)

" The long extract from Professor Humphrey's speech which you give in this evening's *Mail* contains only one point which I shall allude to, because it is one upon which I can speak with authority. 'The man who first employed the carbolic ligature would never have ventured upon it on the human body, had he not first carefully tried it upon animals.' This is just one of the cases where vivisection has led us astray. If the carbolic ligature had never been tried on animals, where it seems to answer admirably, it never would have been tried on human patients, where it fails miserably and has cost many lives. The fact is that the diseases of animals are so different from those of men, wounds in animals act so differently from those of humanity, that the conclusions of vivisections are absolutely worthless. They have done far more harm than good in surgery."—Letter in *Birmingham Daily Mail*, Jan. 21, 1882.

—— A Science Falsely so Called.   Tait.

LAWSON TAIT, F.R.C.S., late Professor of Gynæcology, Queen's College, Birmingham. (A.V.)

" Shortly after I had finished my curriculum, I was fortunate enough to be appointed house-surgeon to a small hospital in Yorkshire, little known outside its own district, but ever likely to keep a strong hold on my affections, founded by John Clayton, in the city of Wakefield. There I had an enormous mass of surgical material at my disposal, and a kindly and indulgent staff, under whose direction I was permitted to make full use of it. Lister had just published his first papers, and had hardly grasped, certainly had not fully formulated, his splendid idea of antiseptic surgery. From 1867 till 1870, Lister had no more faithful disciple, no more devoted follower, than the unknown house-surgeon of the Clayton Hospital. I spent my days with my hands soaked in carbolic oil, making carbolic putty and securing carbolic lac plaster. Compound fractures were saved, which in Edinburgh would have been condemned to amputation, and I did operations successfully, which astonished others as much as they gratified me. Years after, when I had fallen away from the faith, the argument against me, which alone caused me grief, was the assertion that I had never seen and did not understand Listerism. I had been to Glasgow to see it, I had carried it out more scrupulously than the master himself, I had suffered painful attacks of hæmaturia from my misguided enthusiasm years before my metropolitan critics had known what carbolic acid was. But with all my success there occurred the old troubles, death from pyæmia, loss of cases which I could not understand if Lister's doctrines were true. I thought a royal road to surgical success had been opened to me, yet every now and then I found myself floundering out of it, and I began to think it was a science falsely so called."—*From an Address on the Development of Energy and the Germ Theory,* "British Medical Journal," July 23rd, 1887.

ANTISEPTIC SURGERY— Cheyne.
A Science Falsely so Called.

W. WATSON CHEYNE, F.R.C.S., Hunterian Professor, Professor of Surgery, King's College Hospital. (V.)

"It is questionable whether, in the case of wounds which have become septic, it is well to wash them out with irritating antiseptics, as is so often done at present. . . . It has been found that in cases of tubercular disease of joints and bones accompanied by suppuration, general tuberculosis—more especially tubercular meningitis—occurs by far most frequently where the sinuses have become septic, and more especially when, in addition, those septic sinuses have been much irritated by futile antiseptic injections."—*Lectures on Suppuration and Septic Diseases,* " British Medical Journal," March 3rd, 1888, p. 456.

—— The same. Keith.

THOMAS KEITH, M.D., etc., Edinburgh. (V.)

" When I began to use carbolic spray I tried to do without drainage, but for long have gone back to it. For some time I have not found the carbolic spray necessary, and have not used it in my last twenty-seven cases, all of whom have recovered easily. With every possible care the spray has not in my hands prevented the mildest septicæmia, and the effects on the kidney were sometimes disastrous. I have frequently seen kidney hæmorrhage follow long operations, and two deaths in hospital patients were occasioned, I believe, by carbolic acid poisoning."—*Proceedings Inter. Med. Congress,* 1881. Vol. II., p. 236.

—— The same. Lister.

SIR JOSEPH LISTER, Bart., M.D., F.R.S., Consulting Surgeon, King's College Hospital, London. (V.)

"As regards the spray, I feel ashamed that I should have ever recommended it for the purpose of destroying the microbes of the air. If we watch the formation of thes pray and observe how its narrow initial cone expands as it advances, with fresh portions of air continually drawn into its vortex, we see that many of the microbes in it, having only just come under its influence, cannot possibly have been deprived of their vitality. Yet there was a time when I assumed that such was the case. and, trusting the spray implicitly as an atmosphere free from living organisms, omitted various precautions which I had before supposed to be essential."—*Address before the International Medical Congress at Berlin, August,* 1890, *reported in the "British Medical Journal,"* Aug. 16th, 1890, pp. 378-9.

ANTISEPTIC SURGERY. Dott.

D. B. DOTT, Pharmaceutical Chemist, South Canongate, Edinburgh. (V.)

" Other substances which are, or have been. used in the preparation of antiseptic gauze are thymol, 'sanitas,' sal-alembroth, ' sero-sublimate,' and the so-called cyanide of zinc and mercury. The advent of the sero-sublimate was heralded with a good flourish of trumpets, but it seems now to have faded in favour. It is prepared by dissolving corrosive sublimate in the serum of horses' blood, and saturating the gauze therewith. Its value depends on the fact that, in presence of excess of albumen, mercuric chloride to a great extent loses its irritating properties, while still retaining its antiseptic power. From all I can learn, the double cyanide has hardly borne out its early promise, and the perfect antiseptic gauze is still a thing of the future."—*From "Antiseptic Gauze," by D. B. Dott, " Chemist and Druggist,"* Oct. 4th, 1890, p. 487.

APOMORPHIA. Berdoe.

EDWARD BERDOE, M.R.C.S., L.R.C.P.Ed., London. (A.V.)

" This is an alkaloid prepared from morphia. It is used in medicine as an emetic and expectorant. Doctors using this drug for these purposes have found that in young subjects very considerable depression has been produced by it with dangerous symptoms of paralysis of the heart. But Siebert and Moerz, experimenting with the drug upon animals, say that these facts are contradicted by their physiological observations, as they find that apomorphia does not affect the blood pressure, and that the pulse rises when the emetic effect is produced.— *Bartholow's Materia Medica,* p. 459.

" Hypodermic injections of this poison in the lower animals

elicit no evidence of pain, although in man they have been known to cause intense pain.—*Wood*, p. 437.

" Quehl says the paralysis produced by the drug must be central, since neither the sensitive nor motor nerves nor muscles are affected by the poison.—*Ueber die Physiol.*, Halle, 1872.

" Moerz says that during the vomiting the temperature *rises.* —*Wood*, p. 438.

" Harnack, after experimenting upon frogs which he poisoned with apomorphia, after cutting off their legs, directly contradicts Quehl's conclusions.—*Archiv. Exper. Pathol.*, Bd. ii. p. 291.

" Bourgeois declares that in man the drug has *no influence* on the temperature.—*Wood*, p. 438.

" Ziolkowski says the temperature *falls* during the vomiting. —*Ut supra.*"

—*The Futility of Experiments with Drugs on Animals*, by Edward Berdoe (London, 1889), pp. 12, 13.

ARSENIC, Experiments on Frogs with.   Berdoe.

EDWARD BERDOE, M.R.C.S., L.R.C.P.Ed., London.   (A.V.)

" Drs. Ringer and Murrell (*Journal of Physiology*, I. p. 217) experimented upon frogs with arsenic. Dr. W. Sklarck, of Berlin (*Reichert's Archiv*, 1866), experimented in a similar manner with this chemical on the muscular and nervous system of frogs, obtaining very different results from those of the English physiologists. These gentlemen endeavour to extricate physiological medicine from this difficulty by saying that the discrepancies in question depend upon the time of year at which the frogs were experimented upon. We do not dispute that this may materially affect the results, but of what avail is it to study the effects of the medical uses of a drug intended for the treatment of man upon a frog's system which behaves in one manner in spring and a totally different manner in autumn? This confusion illustrates one other of the many fallacies of a system of medicine founded upon any such basis."—*The Futility of Experiments with Drugs on Animals*, by Edward Berdoe (London, 1889), p. 13.

ATROPINE.—See Belladonna.

BELLADONNA (Deadly Nightshade).   Berdoe.

EDWARD BERDOE, M.R.C.S., L.R.C.P.Ed., London.   (A.V.)

" The root and leaves of the poisonous plant *Atropa Belladonna*

contain the alkaloid *Atropina* ; it is entirely to this active principle that the physiological action of Belladonna is due. The
plant and its alkaloid act much more mildly upon the lower
animals than upon man. Its well-known action in dilating the
pupil of the human eye may instructively be compared with its
powerlessness to cause any such effect on the pupils of the eyes
of pigeons, or, as Stillé says, of those of other birds.

" Birds and herbivorous animals eat Belladonna with impunity. ' This is one of the many examples,' say those great
authorities, Drs. Stillé and Maisch, ' which show the danger of
concluding from the lower animals to man in regard to the uses
of medicines, unless the mode of action in the two cases is first
proved to be identical. In no animal is there any degree of
that delirious excitement which Belladonna produces in man.'
—(*Therapeutics*, p. 276.)

" Dr. Ringer (*Materia Medica*, p. 454, 5th ed.) says :—' Certain animals, like pigeons and rabbits, appear to be almost insusceptible to the influence of Belladonna,' and ' Belladonna, it
is asserted, has very little effect on horses and donkeys. So
powerful is the action of atropine on the human organism, that
it is usually medicinally administered in the very minute dose of
from $\frac{1}{130}$ to $\frac{1}{40}$ of a grain. Yet Calmus found that no less than
fifteen grains are required to kill a rabbit, and Ringer says that
two grains administered hypodermically are necessary to kill a
pigeon.

" Meuriot administered atropine to various animals, and then
opened their abdomens whilst alive. He declared that the
poison caused the intestines to undergo violent contraction.

" Bezold and Bloebaum did exactly the same, and they affirm
that they found the poison caused marked sedation (calming)
in the same organs."
—*The Futility of Experiments with Drugs on Animals*, by
Edward Berdoe (London, 1889), p. 14.

BENEFIT TO PRACTICAL MEDICINE. Tait.

LAWSON TAIT, F.R.C.S., late Professor of Gynæcology, Queen's
College, Birmingham. (A.V.)

The Cullen Jubilee Prize given "for the greatest benefit done
to practical medicine by applying surgical means for the relief
of medical cases," and the " Lister Jubilee Prize " given " for
the greatest benefit done to practical surgery in the triennial
period prior to June," 1890, were awarded to Prof. Lawson
Tait, the anti-vivisectionist, by the Colleges of Physicians and
Surgeons of Edinburgh.—*Zoophilist*, Aug. 1st, 1890.

BENZOIC ACID, Contradictory   Berdoe.
Experiments with.

EDWARD BERDOE, M.R.C.S., L.R.C.P.Ed., London. (A.V.)

" Cruel experiments with this drug have been performed by
different physiologists, with the result, says Wood, p. 531,
that their testimony is ‘singularly contradictory.’ "—*The
Futility of Experiments with Drugs on Animals* (London,
1889), p. 15.

BILE, SECRETION OF, Futility of   Tait.
Experiments on Animals as to.

LAWSON TAIT, F.R.C.S., late Professor of Gynæcology, Queen's
    College, Birmingham. (A.V.)

" Whilst watching these cases, I have read much of the
literature of investigations concerning the functions of the bile,
and I have been greatly amused to see how utterly futile experiments on animals have been in settling even the most
elementary facts of the influence and uses of the human bile.
Thus I have not seen the slightest evidence to believe that
either quantity or quality of food, or any drugs which were
used for the legitimate treatment of these cases, as morphia,
calomel, podophyllin, and rhubarb, have the slightest effect on
the quantity and quality of the secretion."—*British Medical
Journal*, May 3rd, 1884.

BLOOD, THE CIRCULATION OF, Harvey and.   Bowie.

JOHN BOWIE, L.R.C.P., L.R.C.S., Edinburgh. (A.V.)

" Various writers on anatomy and physiology were guessing
at the real solution of the problem, but it was the justly re-
nowned Harvey who first reasoned out the fact and enabled
others to see the wonders connected with the circulatory system.
He reasoned out the truth of the circulation from the position,
attachment, and arrangement of the valves of the veins found
in the human body after death. On this point he says, ‘ I was
led to distrust the existing belief of the course of the blood by
considering the arrangement of the valves of the veins. It was
plain that the common doctrine that the blood moved to and
fro in the veins, outwards from the heart, and back again, was
incompatible with the fact of the direction of the valves, which
were so placed that the blood could only move in one direction.’
Now, Harvey in his remarkable little book insists on these
facts as the cause of his discovery. It was on the dead human

body that these were discovered, and not on living animals; therefore experiments on animals cannot be taken into account as having anything to do with the discovery of the circulation of the blood."—*Reply to Dr. Rutherford*, Dec. 14th, 1880 (*Review* Office, 20, St. Giles Street, Edinburgh), p. 7.

BLOOD, THE CIRCULATION OF THE. Harvey.

WILLIAM HARVEY, M.D. (the late), Physician to the King, Prof. of Anatomy and Surgery to the College of Physicians (born 1578 ; died 1657). (V.)

"Speaking of Galen's most meaningless and utterly useless experiment of dividing the trachea of a living dog, forcibly distending the lungs with a pair of bellows, and then tying the trachea securely, he says : ' Who, indeed, doubts that, did he inflate the lungs of a subject in the dissecting-room, he would instantly see the air making its way by this route, were there actually any passage for it ? ' [In this case Harvey was clearly of opinion that vivisection was useless. L. Tait, F.R.C.S.]"—*See "Harvey on the Circulation of the Blood," edited by Dr. A. Bowie* (London, George Bell & Sons, 1889), p. 17.

"This truth, indeed, presents itself obviously before us when we consider what happens in the dissection of living animals ; the great artery need not be divided, but a very small branch only (as Galen even proves in regard to man), to have the whole of the blood in the body, as well that of the veins as of the arteries, drained away in the course of no long time—some half-hour or less. Butchers are well aware of the fact, and can bear witness to it ; for, cutting the throat of an ox and so dividing the vessels of the neck, in less than a quarter of an hour they have all the vessels bloodless. The same thing also occasionally occurs with great rapidity in performing amputations and removing tumours in the human subject." ["Here vivisection experiment was therefore wholly unnecessary, but Harvey did not see it." L. Tait.]—*The same book*, p. 53.

"The internal jugular vein of a live fallow deer having been exposed (many of the nobility and his most serene Majesty the King, my master, being present), was divided, but a few drops of blood were observed to escape from the lower orifice rising up from under the clavicle : whilst from the superior orifice of the vein, and coming down from the head, a round torrent of blood gushed forth. You may observe the same fact any day in practising phlebotomy : if with a finger you compress the vein a little below the orifice, the blood is immediately arrested ; but the pressure being removed, forthwith the flow returns as before."—*The same book (as above)*, p. 131. ["The experiment on the stag alluded to here forms, so far as I can discover, the basis of Hannay's well-known picture, which affords the British public the proof of Harvey's claim as the discoverer of the circulation, very much as popular theology is drawn from Milton's 'Paradise Lost.' But Harvey admits in the last sentence that the experiment was wholly unnecessary."— *Lawson Tait, F.R.C.S. " Uselessness of Vivisection," New Ed.*, 1883, pp. 9-11 note.]

BLOOD, THE CIRCULATION OF THE.   Harvey.

WILLIAM HARVEY, M.D. (the late), Physician to the King, Prof. of Anatomy and Surgery to the College of Physicians (born 1578; died 1657.) (V.)

" And sooth to say, when I surveyed my mass of evidence, whether derived from vivisections, and my various reflections on them, or from the ventricles of the heart, and the vessels that enter into and issue from them, the symmetry and size of these conduits,—for nature doing nothing in vain, would never have given them so large a relative size without a purpose,—or from the arrangement and intimate structure of the valves in particular, and of the other parts of the heart in general, with many things besides, I frequently and seriously bethought me, and long revolved in my mind, what might be the quantity of blood which was transmitted, in how short a time its passage might be effected, and the like. *But not finding it possible that this could be supplied by the juices of the ingested aliment, without the veins on the one hand becoming drained, and the arteries on the other getting ruptured through the excessive charge of blood, unless the blood should somehow find its way from the arteries into the veins,* and so return to the right side of the heart ; I began to think whether there might not be A MOTION, AS IT WERE, IN A CIRCLE. Now this I afterwards found to be true ; and I finally saw that the blood, forced by the action of the left ventricle into the arteries, was distributed to the body at large, and its several parts, *in the same manner as it is sent through the lungs*, impelled by the right ventricle into the pulmonary artery, and that it then passed through the veins, and along the *vena cava*, and so round to the left ventricle in the manner already indicated."—*Harvey on the Circulation of the Blood, edited by Dr. A. Bowie* (London, George Bell & Sons, 1889), p. 48.

BLOOD, THE CIRCULATION OF THE. Harvey.

WILLIAM HARVEY, M.D. (the late), Physician to the King, Prof.
of Anatomy and Surgery to the College of Physicians (born 1578;
died 1657). (V.)

"It may be well here to relate an experiment which I lately
tried in the presence of several of my colleagues. . . .
Having tied the pulmonary artery, the pulmonary veins, and
the aorta, in the body of a man who had been hanged. and then
opened the left ventricle of the heart, we passed a tube through
the *vena cava* into the right ventricle of the heart, and having.
at the same time, attached an ox's bladder to the tube, . . .
we filled it nearly full of warm water, and forcibly injected the
fluid into the heart, so that the greater part of a pound of water
was thrown into the right auricle and ventricle. The result was
that the right auricle and ventricle were enormously distended.
but not a drop of water or of blood made its escape through
the orifice in the left ventricle. The ligatures having been un-
done, the same tube was passed into the pulmonary artery, and
a tight ligature having been put round it to prevent any reflux
into the right ventricle, the water in the bladder was now
pushed towards the lungs, upon which a torrent of the fluid,
mixed with a quantity of blood. immediately gushed forth from
the perforation in the left ventricle; so that a quantity of
water, equal to that which was pressed from the bladder into
the lungs at each effort, instantly escaped by the perforation
mentioned."—*Dr. Willis's Edition of "The Life and Works of
William Harvey"* (Sydenham Society), p. 507.

—— The same. Macilwain.

GEORGE MACILWAIN, F.R.C.S. (the late), a witness before the
Royal Commission, 1875 (born 1797; died 1882). (A.V.)

"I find that the discovery of the circulation of the blood
is referred to vivisection. In the first place, any man who
knows what the circulation is will see that intrinsically
that could not be; you do not want the authority which is
suggested to you. because you could not discover the circulation
in the living body; I do not see how it is possible to do it.
If you had a dead body, then it is so easy to discover the
circulation that it is difficult to understand how it was not done
before; because if you inject by the arteries you find that it is
returned by the veins. Harvey was a pupil of Fabricius of
Aqua Pendente, and Fabricius discovered the valves in the
superficial veins. Of course the blood can only move in one
direction, but Fabricius did not see that. Harvey did; and

E

that is the real seed of his discovery. But you see it said every day, and I see medical men say, it was from vivisection —from experiments, at least, on living animals."—*Evid. Roy. Com.* (London, 1876), Q. 1845-6.

BLOOD, THE CIRCULATION OF THE.   Tait.

LAWSON TAIT, F.R.C.S., late Professor of Gynæcology, Queen's College, Birmingham. (A.V.)

" Take the case of the alleged discovery of the circulation of the blood by Harvey, and it can be clearly shown that quite as much as Harvey knew was known before his time, and that it is only our insular pride which has claimed for him the merit of the discovery. That he made any solid contribution to the facts of the case by vivisection is conclusively disproved, and this was practically admitted before the Commission by such good authorities as Dr. Acland and Dr. Lauder Brunton. The circulation was not proved till Malpighi used the microscope, and though in that observation he used a vivisectional experiment, his proceeding was wholly unnecessary, for he could have better and more easily have used the web of the frog's foot than its lung. It is, moreover, perfectly clear that were it incumbent on any one to prove the circulation of the blood now as a new theme, it could not be done by any vivisectional process, but could at once be satisfactorily established by a dead body and an injecting syringe. In fact, I think I might almost say that the systemic circulation remained incompletely proved until the examination of injected tissues by the micro. scope had been made."—" *The Uselessness of Vivisection,*" *a paper read before the Birmingham Philosophical Society, April* 20, 1882 (*New Ed.* 1883, pp. 3, 4).

BLOOD PRESSURE, Experiments as to.   Macaulay.

JAMES MACAULAY, M.A., M.D., F.R.C.S.Ed., London. (A.V.)

" As to the experiments on the statics and dynamics of the circulation, from those of Hales to those of Ludwig, no doubt many facts have been ascertained and recorded, as is the case with all experiments, but no new or practical results appear ' for the benefit of humanity.' As to the absolute force of the heart considered as a hydraulic machine, and the velocity of the blood, the results of experiment vary much, and those of old Stephen Hales give probably as near an average estimate as can be expected. But for practical application in medicine the numerous experiments made since the time of Hales are quite useless. The force of the heart, for example, varies in the animals inspected, and under different conditions ; and the variations are infinite in different persons, in various conditions of age, strength, and state of health. The general estimates may be interesting as facts for philosophical statement, but are useless with any view of applying such experiments to use, in maladies either of the sanguineous or nervous system. More useful information can be obtained by observing the force of the heart as indicated on the delicate dial of a balance chair, than from all the experiments of vivisectors."—" *Vivisection*," *A Prize Essay* (London, 1881), p. 41.

BONE GRAFTING.—*See* PAINFUL EXPERIMENTS.

BONE GROWTH—Function of the Periosteum. Tait.

LAWSON TAIT, F.R.C.S., late Professor of Gynæcology, Queen's College, Birmingham. (A.V.)

" The history of the development of our knowledge of the formation and growth of bone is extremely interesting, because it shows how completely misleading are the conclusions based upon vivisectional experiments, and how perfectly the secrets of Nature may be unravelled by a careful and intelligent examination of her own experiments. No one can look now at a necrosed bone without seeing how completely the whole story is there written. The history also exemplifies the fact that it is not only the purely practical details of surgery which are independent of vivisection for their development, but what are called the more scientific developments of physiological knowledge are equally possible without its aid, and are often retarded by its misguidance. . . . Between 1739 and 1743 Henri Louis Duhamel-Dumonceau published eight memoirs on the growth and repair of bones, largely based on the suggestive discovery of Belchier. Up to this time the formation of callus was thought to be due to an effusion of osseous juice—a belief which pervaded the surgical teaching of a distinguished professor of the University of Edinburgh so late as my own student days—but Duhamel proved its real origin. He also completely established the fact that bones grow in thickness by the addition of osseous layers originating from the periosteum. . . . Mr. Goodsir's conclusions are, on the contrary, uniformly accepted, and as to his method he says that they were made upon shafts of human bones which had died,—museum specimens, just as Duhamel's were. They showed that whilst the periosteum is the matrix and

machine by which the new bone is made, the real agency
is in the layer of osteal cells, and so he finally solved the
riddle. He did this by microscopic and pathological research.
He condemned the employment of vivisection as useless and
misleading, and to him we owe the completion of Belchier's
and Duhamel's research—a completion which was hindered for
a century by the blunders of vivisectionists."—" *Uselessness
of Vivisection*," by Lawson Tait (Birmingham. 1882). pp. 28,
30–33.

BOREL ON CRUELTY.—*See* CRUELTY OF VIVISECTION.

BOY AND DOG UNITED.—*See* PAINFUL EXPERIMENTS.

BRAIN, The.   Brown Séquard.

CHARLES ÉDOUARD BROWN-SÉQUARD (the late), Professor
   of Experimental Medicine at the College of France. (V.)

   " The danger of making use of experiments on living animals
exclusively is very strikingly illustrated by the many errors
concerning the cerebellum committed by experimental physiologists, who mistook the effects of certain circumstances
of their experiments for the results of injuries or of the
absence of the cerebellum. Had they taken the trouble
of comparing the phenomena they saw with those observed by
medical men in cases of disease of the cerebellum, they would
not have introduced in science a number of hypotheses which
impede its progress."—*The Lancet*, vol. ii. 1858, p. 1.

—— The same.   " The Lancet."

" THE LANCET," London. (V.)

   " It is an interesting and noteworthy fact that pathological
observation is doing more to advance our knowledge of cerebral
functions than physiological experiment. At any rate this
would seem to be true of the doctrine of cerebral localization,
for whereas the physiologists agree to differ upon the interpretation of their experimental results in this matter, the clinical
and pathological evidence in support of the doctrine is rapidly
accumulating."—*Lancet*, June 16th, 1883.

—— The same.   Macaulay.

JAMES MACAULAY, M.A., M.D., F.R.C.S.Ed., London.   (A.V.)

   " With regard to the alleged discovery of the functions of the
several parts of the encephalon, to the experimental investiga-

tions of which some hundreds of physiologists have devoted much labour, there are very few results universally accepted. If we include articles and reports in medical and scientific journals, as well as treatises separately published, we have a huge library describing such investigations, but the conclusions arrived at would not fill one octavo page. There is not a subject in the whole range of research about which there are so many vague and so many contradictory statements. The most recent experimenters seem to be going over the same dreary and dismal ground as their predecessors.—" *Vivisection*,".*A Prize Essay* (London, 1881), page 40.

BRAIN, The.   Marvaud.

DR. MARVAUD, Paris. (V.)

" It is impossible to wound the head and open the skull without causing a severe shock to the system of the animals, and a more or less violent irritation of the brain ; that is to say, not without producing a certain amount of pain. And we know the influence that pain can have, not only on the functions of the great organic apparatus (circulation, respiration, animal heat). but also on the anatomical and physiological state of the nerve centres."—DR. MARVAUD, *Gazette Médicale de Paris*, 1878 (pp. 81, 82).

—— The same.   Hall.

RADCLIFFE HALL, M.D. (the late) Edinburgh. (V.)

" This author, in speaking of the ganglion of the sympathetic connected with the fifth nerve, and known as the ophthalmic or ciliary, says, ' in the rabbit, the iris receives fibres from the sixth pair which do not pass through the ganglion ; and it is through this that the contraction of the pupil is produced in that animal by irritation of the fifth pair, which will not produce any effect upon the pupil of the dog, cat or pigeon, so long as it does not affect the brain to the extent of producing vertigo, nor affect the visual sense in any other way.'"—*Edinburgh Med. and Surg. Jour.* (1846-8).

—— The same.   Tait.

LAWSON TAIT, F.R.C.S., late Professor of Gynæcology, Queen's College, Birmingham. (A.V.)

" Mr. Gamgee tells us that the *Académie de Chirurgie* gave

out the subject of Contre-coup* and its influence in injuries of the
head as a subject for a prize competition, and that the prize
was obtained in 1778 by M. Saucerotte, whose essay was based
'on literary research, clinical observations, and twenty-one
experiments on living dogs.' He omits, however, to make any
estimate of the value of the experiments on the dogs, which
seems to me to be absolutely nothing ; and he quite forgets to
mention that the theory of contre-coup had been completely
established for nearly two centuries before, and had been
particularly the subject of Paul Ammannus of Leipsic, who
wrote a well-known work, ' *De resonitu seu contra fissura
cranii*,' in 1674, in which trepanning is recommended at the
point of contre-coup, as had been practised by Paul Barbette,
of Amsterdam, thirteen years before that. The theory of contre-
coup and the fatal practices arising from it are happily now
buried in oblivion in spite of Saucerotte's vivisection, and
would never again have been alluded to but for Mr. Gamgee's
unfortunate resurrection of them. The modern verdict concerning fractures of the skull is given tersely in Mr. Flint
South's words, 'the less done as regards meddling with them
the better,' and 'a knowledge of counter-fractures is quite
uncertain.' In fact, nothing could be more unfortunate than
the selection of M. Saucerotte's experiments as an illustration
of the value of vivisection, for they were performed for a purpose which was long ago recognised as futile, and in support
of a practice universally condemned.

⁂   ⁂   ⁂   ⁂

" Reading his (Saucerotte's) experiments, they seem so like
Ferrier's that I fancy if Dr. Ferrier had known of the existence
of this essay he would have found little need to repeat its work."
—" *Uselessness of Vivisection* " (*Birmingham Philosophical
Society*, 1882), pp. 13, 15.

BRAIN, The.   Blackwood.

WILLIAM BLACKWOOD, M.D., Philadelphia, U.S.A. (A.V.)

" I deny that our present knowledge of nervous brain disease
is due at all to the work of vivisectors, and affirm that vivisectors are less capable of managing such diseases than
ordinarily intelligent physicians. . . . The foundation for
vivisection is wrong, the conclusions cannot be true."—*Address
at Philadelphia*, 1885.

---

* Contre-coup is a concussion or shock produced by a blow or other injury,
in a part or region opposite to that at which the blow is received often causing
rupture or disorganization of the parts affected.—*Webster's Dict.*, Ed. 1890.

BRAIN, The.   Elliotson.

JOHN ELLIOTSON, M.D. (the late), Professor of the Practice of
    Medicine, University of London (born 1791 ; died 1868). (V.)

" I once enjoyed an opportunity of very distinctly observing
the motions of the brain, and making some experiments with
respect to it.   A young man eighteen years old, had five years
previously fallen from an eminence and fractured the frontal
bone on the left side of the coronal suture, since which time
there had been an immense hiatus, covered by merely a soft
cicatrix, and the common integuments.

          ⁜   ⁜   ⁜   ⁜   ⁜

" I may add that this wound on the *left* side of the head had
rendered the right arm and leg paralytic."—*Physiology*, p. 341,
note.

[" Morgagni gives a case of cerebral lesion (separation of the
corpus striatum from the cortex) which he had carefully
observed and examined *post-mortem*.   He was astonished to
find paralysis apparently on the same side as the lesion ; but
distrusting his recollection and the accuracy of his records, he
asked of his students, on which side the paralysis had existed.
' All in general and each one in particular answered without
hesitation that it was the right side (the side of the disease) ;
and for this reason,' said he, ' it is clear to me that *sometimes*
the paralysis occurs on the same side as the lesion.' "—*Ferrier*.]

—— The same.   Ferrier.

DAVID FERRIER, M.D., F.R.S., Professor of Neuropathy, King's
    College, London.   (V.)

" Moreover, the degrees of evolution of the central nervous
system, from the simplest reflex mechanism up to the highest
encephalic centres according as we ascend or descend the
animal scale, introduce other complications, and render the
application of the results of experiment on the brain of a frog,
or a pigeon, or a rabbit, without due qualification, to the physiology of the human brain, very questionable : or even lead to
conclusions seriously at variance with well-established facts of
clinical and pathological observation.

          ⁜   ⁜   ⁜   ⁜

" No one who has attentively studied the results of the labours
of the numerous investigators in this field of research, can help
being struck by the want of harmony, and even positive contradictions, among the conclusions which apparently the same
experiments and the same facts have led to in different hands."
—*Ferrier's " Functions of the Brain,"* Preface.

BRAIN, The.   Charcot.

JEAN M. CHARCOT, M.D. (the late), Physician to the Salpetrière
Hospital, Paris (born 1825 ; died 1893). (V.)

" Experimentation with animals that are nearest to man—still
more with those far removed from man in the zoological scale—
cannot, however faultless its technique, however definite its
results, solve finally the problems raised by the pathology of
the human brain. In brain it is, above all, that we differ from
animals. That organ attains in man a degree of development
and of perfection not reached in any other species. Its functions become complex, while at the same time its morphology
undergoes important modifications. Now, it is perfectly clear
that as regards questions of localization, morphological details
are of the first importance. As for functions, even if we take
account only of those common to men and animals, they are
not performed in all in the same way. The higher an organism
stands in the animal scale, the more strictly are the purely reflex
functions subordinated to the functions of the higher centres.
A decapitated frog performs with its legs co-ordinated automatic
movements : not so a decapitated dog. In the dog, brain
lesions, even of considerable extent, produce only incomplete
paralysis, often passing away, while in man the like lesions
cause incurable functional troubles. These examples are
enough to show that, particularly as regards brain functions,
the utmost reserve is necessary in drawing inferences from
animals to man. The results of experimentation, however
ingenious, however skilfully conducted, can give only presump-
tions more or less strong, but never absolute demonstration."—
*Prof. Charcot, on " The Topography of the Brain," in " The
Forum* " (New York, U.S.A.), August, 1888, pp. 615-616.

—— The same.   Charcot.

JEAN M. CHARCOT, M.D. (the late), Physician to the Salpetrière
Hospital, Paris (born 1825 ; died 1893). (V.)

" Hence, the only really decisive *data* touching the cerebral
pathology of man are, in my opinion, those developed according
to the principles of the anatomo-clinical method. That method
consists in ever confronting the functional disorders observed
during life with the lesions discovered and carefully located
after death. This is the method which enabled Laennec to
throw light on the difficult subject of diagnosing pulmonary
affections, and it has also materially helped the diagnosis of
diseases of the liver, kidneys and spinal cord. To it, I may
justly say, we owe whatever definite knowledge we have of brain

pathology. As for the localization of certain cerebral functions, this method is not only the best, but the only one that can be employed. What light, for instance. could experimentation [on animals] have thrown upon the question as to the seat of the functions of speech—functions which are special to man?" —*From " The Topography of the Brain." By Professor Charcot, in " The Forum"* (New York, U.S.A.), August 1888, p. 616.

BRAIN, The. Ferrier.

DAVID FERRIER, M.D., F.R.S., Professor of Neuropathy, King's College, London. (V.)

" He reviewed the difficulties attending the introduction of cerebral surgery. There was a great future before it. but care must be taken not to overdo it. Septic infection was not the only danger. He had seen several unsuccessful operations and deaths, though recoveries predominated. . . . He was disappointed in the results in Jacksonian epilepsy and discharging irritative lesions of the cortex. There had been relapses, and in some cases the cure of the epilepsy left a worse state— hemiplegia and loss of speech."—*From Summary of Prof. Ferrier's Speech at the first Triennial Congress of American Physicians and Surgeons, Washington, Sept. 18-25, 1888 ; reported in " The British Medical Journal,"* Nov. 3, 1888.

—— The same. Horsley.

VICTOR HORSLEY, M.B., F.R.S., Professor of Pathology, University College, London. (V.)

" He advocated early operation. It required much courage, for the operation was always attended with liability to death of the patient. When the epilepsy returned, he believed it was on account of incomplete removal of the diseased area, and of a rim of surrounding cells, at least one centimetre in thickness. He was alive to the danger of overdoing in certain cases, but also thought there was considerable danger of our being unduly influenced in our opinions by statistics."—*From Summary of Prof. Horsley's Speech at the first Triennial Congress of American Physicians and Surgeons, Washington. Sept. 18-25, 1888 ; reported in " The British Medical Journal,"* Nov. 3, 1888.

—— The same. Laborde.

J. V. LABORDE, Professor of Practical Physiology, Faculty of Medicine, Paris. (V.)

" By the side of the physiological school, another has sprung up, the researches of which are of far greater utility. I mean the clinical school. . . . If the principles of the clinical school did not themselves speak loudly in its favour, it would be sufficient to cast an eye over the progress made under its guidance to be entirely convinced how great are the legitimate hopes to be conceived therefrom.

　　　※　　　　　　　　※　　　　　　　　※　　　　　　　　　　　　　　　　　※

" The first victory of science over the impenetrable mysteries of the nerve functions, that most brilliant victory, the discovery of the exact seat of aphasia, is the result of clinical practice, which alone could accomplish it.

　　　※　　　　　　　　※　　　　　　　　※　　　　　　　　※　　　　　　　　※

" When that organ is in question, the perfection of which characterizes the highest animal superiority, the brain, to which have been confided the functions of intelligence, of thought. of memory, which in reality make man what he is . . . the study of this organ to bear fruit must be made on man."—*Travaux du Laboratoire de Physiologie, J. V. Laborde*, vol. i. (1885), pp. 55–56.

BRAIN, The. Althaus.

JULIUS ALTHAUS, M.D.Berlin, M.R.C.S.Lond., Consulting Physician, Hospital for Epilepsy and Paralysis, Regent's Park. (P. V.)

" Our systematic handbooks of anatomy do not as yet supply that kind of knowledge which is so much required for a due appreciation of recent medical doctrines, and which has been gained not so much by systematic slicings of brains and cords of healthy adults as by the infinitely finer and more instructive dissections made for us by disease, and which have thrown an entirely new light on the facts of normal anatomy. This is a kind of vivisection which cannot be prohibited by Acts of Parliament. and which has led to far more reliable results than experimental physiology or pathology."—*From a Lecture by Dr. Julius Althaus, " British Medical Journal,"* June 4th, 1881.

BRAIN SURGERY. "F.R.S."

" F.R.S.," the signature adopted by a correspondent of *The Times* newspaper, of London. (V.)

" While the Bishop of Oxford and Professor Ruskin were, on somewhat intangible grounds, denouncing vivisection at Oxford last Tuesday afternoon, there sat at one of the windows of the

Hospital for Epilepsy and Paralysis, in Regent's Park, in an invalid chair, propped up with pillows, pale and careworn, but with a hopeful smile on his face, a man who could have spoken a really pertinent word upon the subject, and told the right rev. prelate and great art critic that he owed his life, and his wife and children their rescue from bereavement and penury, to some of these experiments on living animals which they so roundly condemned.

*   *   *   *   *

" This case—this impressive and illustrative case—is that of a man who, when admitted to the Hospital for Epilepsy and Paralysis, presented a group of symptoms which pointed to tumour of the brain—a distressing and hitherto necessarily fatal malady, for the diagnosis or recognition of which we are indebted to bed-side experience and *post-mortem* examination. But while clinical and pathological observations have supplied us with knowledge which enables us to detect the existence of tumours of the brain, they have not afforded us any clue to the situation of these morbid growths in the brain-mass, and it was not until Professor Ferrier had, by his experiments on animals, demonstrated the localization of sensory and motor functions in the cerebral hemispheres that the position of any diseased process by which they might be invaded could be definitely determined. By the light of these experiments it is now possible in many instances to map out the seat of certain pathological changes in these hemispheres with as much nicety and certainty as if the skull and its coverings and linings had become transparent, so that the surface of the brain was exposed to direct inspection. And thus in the case to which I am referring, Dr. Hughes Bennett, under whose care the patient was, guided by Ferrier's experiments, skilfully interpreted the palsies and convulsive movements which the man exhibited, and deduced from them that a small tumour was lodged at one particular point in his ' dome of thought,' and was silently and relentlessly eating its way into surrounding textures.

*   *   *

"On the 25th ultimo accordingly, Mr. Godlee, surgeon to University College Hospital, in the midst of an earnest and anxious band of medical men, made an opening in the scalp, skull, and brain membranes of this man at the point where Dr. Hughes Bennett had placed his divining finger, the point corresponding with the convolution where he declared the peccant body to be, and where sure enough it was discovered. In the substance of the brain, exactly where Dr. Hughes Bennett had predicted, a tumour the size of a walnut was found—a tumour which Mr. Godlee removed without difficulty. The man is now convalescent, having never had a bad symptom, and full of gratitude for the relief afforded him. He has been snatched from the grave."—*Extracts from letter in "The Times,"* Dec. 16th, 1884.

BRAIN SURGERY. "F.R.S."

"F.R.S." the signature adopted by a correspondent of *The Times* newspaper, of London. (V.)

"Intelligence has just reached me that the man from whom the tumour was removed, and who was regarded as convalescent, died unexpectedly on Tuesday last, exactly four weeks after the operation, from one of those complications by which any surgical operation may be attended. An eminent surgeon who is not on the staff of the hospital, but who was led by his interest in the case to visit and examine the man, pronounced him, as late as the 16th inst., in a completely satisfactory condition ; but subsequently a change for the worse took place, and he passed away on the 23rd inst."—*Letter in "The Times,"* Dec. 26th, 1884.

—— Successful cases without Vivisection. Whitson.

JAMES WHITSON, M.B. and C.M., Lecturer on Operative Surgery, St. Mungo's College, Glasgow. (V.)

"Your correspondent is, however, in error in imagining that the case described by him is either unique, or the first in which the brain has been opened for the removal of tumours or other morbid material. During the last eight years a series of observations have been conducted in the Glasgow Royal Infirmary with the object of localising brain function, and numerous operations have been undertaken within its precincts for the relief of various cerebral diseases.

*   *   *   *   *

"In 1879 three cases came under the care of Dr. Macewen in which the skull was trephined. Two were for injury. The third was performed for the relief of pressure within the skull. The patient had been seized with a form of epilepsy, and while she was plunged in a state of complete coma, with her vitality ebbing rapidly away, Dr. Macewen made an opening through the skull at a particular point and found a tumour of considerable magnitude encroaching on the brain. After a prolonged and troublesome operation every vestige of the growth was removed, and with its extirpation consciousness speedily returned, though a temporary paralysis of the arm and leg still remained. These latter complications, however, subsequently disappeared, and the patient has been constantly at work since she left the hospital. In another case, also affected with epileptoid seizures, the skull was opened, the brain membranes incised, and a considerable quantity of blood which had been poured out and proved to be the cause of the mischief was allowed to escape. A marked clearing of the intellectual faculties was immediately apparent, and convalescence was afterwards fully established.

     *   *   *   *   *

" It is but right to state that since 1879 a number of equally grave cases have been operated on by Dr. Macewen, several of which were shown at a recent demonstration given in the Royal Infirmary."—*Letter of Dr. Whitson in " The Times,"* Dec. 26th, 1884.

BRAIN SURGERY. Whitson.

JAMES WHITSON, M.B. and C.M. Lecturer on Operative Surgery, St. Mungo's College, Glasgow. (V.)

" The statements made in my previous letter may be summarized as follows:—

" 1. The position of cerebral lesions has been accurately localized, and in some cases from motor symptoms alone.

" 2. With a diagnosis of this kind before us, the skull has been opened, the brain cut into, and the nocuous—or, as ' F.R.S.' happily terms it, the peccant—matter removed therefrom.

" 3. These operations have been performed antiseptically.

" 4. The majority have been followed with complete success, the patients being now, not only alive, but among the breadwinners of the present day.

" 5. Therefore the new era in the domain of cerebral surgery narrated by ' F.R.S.,' though only dawning in London within the last few months, has been for years an accomplished fact in Glasgow."—*Letter in " The Times,"* Jan. 3rd, 1885.

—— The same. Goodhart.

JAMES FREDERICK GOODHART, M.D., Physician at Guy's Hospital, London. (V.)

" Unfortunately for ' F.R.S.' 's view, ' says Dr. Goodhart in the Pathological Society's *Transactions*, " I had in my mind

another case in which, according to the diagnostic skill of Dr.
Ferrier himself, a cerebral tumour was judged to be a fit case
for the attempt at its removal. The man died before the
attempt was consummated, and the tumour was found to
occupy the entire thickness of the anterior third of the
affected hemisphere. *This is the way in which* (italics the
Medical Press's) most of these cases reject the advances of surgery."
—*Medical Press*, Jan. 26th, 1887.

BRAIN SURGERY.   Goodhart.

JAMES FREDERICK GOODHART, M.D., M.R.C.S., Physician
    at Guy's Hospital, London.   (V.)

" Dr. Goodhart went on to say that in thirteen years of
post-mortem work he did not remember seeing a single case in
which the tumour was at once accessible and capable of being
localized. This naturally made him doubt the soundness of
' F.R.S.''s judgment, and strongly inclined to take the opposite
view, namely, ' that it is very doubtful whether in the region
of cerebral tumours, other than inflammatory, surgery has any
future worth mention before it.' The *Medical Press* thinks that
if such a case, proving fatal, were brought before a jury, the
latter could not but give a verdict against the surgeon who
operated. Out of fifty-four cases tabulated by the Morbid
Growths Committee of the Pathological Society, only two
seemed suitable for operation ; and the Committee reported
almost in the words of Charcot and Pitres that the symptoms
occasioned by brain tumours were of such an uncertain nature
as to ' very often render their localisation a matter of pure
conjecture.' "—*Medical Press*, Jan. 25th, 1887.

—— The same.   Haughton.

EDWARD HAUGHTON, M.D., M.R.C.S., Spring Grove House,
    Upper Norwood, London. (A.V.)

" Without meaning to depreciate the scientific ability of
those gentlemen who think it wise to trephine the skull in
search of tumours without further guide than the lines laid
down by Professor Ferrier, I cannot think that they have really
established anything new in the vivisection controversy. The
small successes of operations of this kind (even when performed
upon perfectly healthy men who have met with accident
causing depressions of bony spiculæ) would prevent the possibility of any very striking practical results. If only one in
three survives when the operation is performed on healthy
persons, the proportion will evidently be smaller when cerebral

tumours are in question, and the number of cases suitable for operation would also be comparatively small ; so that, as yet, vivisection wants better proof of its practical value to set off against the horrors with which the public have already been made familiar."—*Letter in " The Times,"* Dec. 29th, 1884.

BRAIN. Hermann.

LUDIMAR HERMANN, Professor of Physiology and Medical Physics, Zurich University. (V.)

" Our experiments were intended to decide how far the objection raised on several sides was justified, that the results of the experiments made by Fritsch and Hitzig on the cortex of the cerebrum did not arise from the excitation of the cortex itself, but of the more internal parts. . . . The experiments were made during the summer term of 1874, all on middle-sized dogs, and were carried out successfully. . . . There were only six : as the results were all the same, there was no reason to make more of these cruel experiments. . . . I conclude with the remark that the experiments of Fritsch and Hitzig, however interesting and precious they may be, do not justify any conclusions concerning the functions of the cortex."—" *Ueber elektrische Reizversuche an der Grosshirnrinde,*" *Pflüger's Archiv,* vol. x. pp. 78-84.

—— The same. Hermann.

LUDIMAR HERMANN, Professor of Physiology and Medical Physics, Zurich University. (V.)

" Physiological experiments conducted in these regions are most indefinite. The usual plan of investigation, viz. that of applying stimuli to the brain substance, leads either to negative results, or, if electrical stimulation is used, to results which, owing to the unavoidable dispersal of the currents in numerous directions, are not sufficiently localised to form the basis for trustworthy conclusions. In place of exact observations after section and stimulation of different regions, we have here the far less refined method of observation after lesions—lesions induced in the most delicate and complicated organ of the body by means so absurdly rough that, as Ludwig has forcibly put it, they may be compared to injuries to a watch by means of a pistol-shot. The results obtained in this way are attributable to the most diverse causes ; for, apart from the fact that it is impossible to localise the lesion itself, the results may be due to irritation of centres, paralysis of centres, stimulation of conducting apparatus, or paralysis of conducting apparatus,

without our being able to say which.   Hence the interpretation
of even those phenomena which are constant in their occurrence
is always uncertain.   The third and best method of investigation which is possible is the observation of cases of disease in
which the exact nature of the lesions is accurately ascertained
after death."—*Hermann's Human Physiology*, translated by
Professor Gamgee (London, 1878), p. 444.

BRAIN LOCALISATION—Liability to   Kingsford.
Error and Misconception.

ANNA KINGSFORD, M.D., Paris (the late).   (A.V.)

" The conditions under which experimenters are compelled
to work render their results liable to great misconception and
error.   Thus, in order to reach special tracts and areas of the
brain, they are forced to push their instruments—whether
heated or otherwise—through the superficial membranes and
tissues of the hemispheres lying beneath the skull, and by
these acts of laceration or denudation many complications are
set up which often seriously interfere with the conclusions
sought, making it difficult to determine what proportion of the
results obtained may be due to secondary and unavoidable
injuries."—*Illustrated Science Monthly*, February, 1884.

—— The same.   Kingsford.

ANNA KINGSFORD, M.D., Paris (the late).   (A.V.)

" Professor Charcot points out, in his ' *Leçons sur les Localis-
ations dans les Maladies Cérébrales*.' that the utmost that can be
learned from experiment on the brains of animals is the topography of the animal brain, and that it must still remain for the
science of human anatomy and clinical investigation to
enlighten us in regard to the far more complex and highly
differentiated nervous organization of our own species.   And,
in fact, it is in the department of clinical and *post-mortem* study
that, so far, all our best data for brain localisation have been
secured.   Painstaking and thoughtful observers of cerebral
disease in man were actively and fruitfully at work in this
direction more than ten years before the experimenters had
sacrificed a single animal to the quest.   It has been repeatedly
pointed out by those who are best qualified to judge, that
nature continually presents us with ready-made experiments of
the most delicate and suggestive kind, impossible for mechanical
artifice to realize, on account of the conditions under which
artifice must necessarily work."—*Illustrated Science Monthly*,
February, 1884.

BRAIN LOCALISATION.   " The Lancet."

" THE LANCET," Strand, London.   (V.)

" It must be confessed that the aid ' localisation' has afforded to treatment has been small and practically confined to cases of surgical interference.   Even of these cases there are very few—scarcely more than could be counted on the fingers of the hand—in which the power of localising cerebral disease can be said to have been the means of saving a life that would have been lost without it.   Nor is any clear indication to be seen that such cases are likely to be more frequent.   Very few will share Dr. Ferrier's confident anticipation that the history of abdominal surgery is likely to find a parallel in surgical achievements within the cranial cavity, in spite of the authority with which he cites his experience with the lower animals. . . . If Dr. Ferrier's suggestions meet with much practical response, it is to be feared that cerebral localisation will soon have more deaths to answer for than lives to boast of."—*The Lancet*, Nov. 10th, 1883, p. 823.

BROMIDES OF POTASSIUM,   Berdoe.
AMMONIA, SODIUM, etc.

EDWARD BERDOE, M.R.C.S., L.R.C.P.Ed., London.   (A.V.)

" Bartholow, Purser, and Laborde experimented with the bromides upon the nervous system of different animals, and arrived at certain conclusions, which were promptly contradicted by Darmourette and Polvette, after a similar series of experiments.—(*Wood, Therapeutics*, p. 325)."—*The Futility of Experiments with Drugs on Animals*, by Edward Berdoe (London, 1889), p. 15.

CAFFEIN, Contradictory Experiments with.   Berdoe.

EDWARD BERDOE, M.R.C.S., L.R.C.P.Ed., London.   (A.V.)

" Caffein is prepared from coffee.   Much diversity of opinion exists amongst physiologists as to the action of this drug.   A great number of animals have undergone experiments with it, causing violent spasms, convulsions, and excitement, ending in death.   Dr. Mary P. Jacobi experimented with this potent alkaloid *on a patient whose brain was exposed*. (See *Stillé's Therapeutics*, p. 312.)   Those who experiment with it on frogs note a different action when they use different species of these animals, the action on *rana esculenta* being very different from that on *rana temoraria*—(*Lauder Brunton, Materia Medica*, p. 72.)."—*Ibid*, pp. 15, 16.

F

CALABAR BEAN, Contradictory Experi-   Berdoe.
ments with.

EDWARD BERDOE, M.R.C.S., L.R.C.P.Ed., London. (A.V.)

"This bean is the dried seed of *Physostigma venenosum.*
Bartholow and Bourneville experimented with Calabar bean,
and arrived at conclusions opposite to each other. Indeed, the
most conflicting testimony is given by different physiologists as
to its action on men and animals. Wood (*Therapeutics*, p. 310)
says:—' The researches of Köhler, of Vintschgau, and of
Rossbach and Frohlich, are especially open to doubt, on
account of their statement that Calabar bean tetanizes.' In
summing up the evidence of various vivisectors as to its action
upon the vagi nerves, it appears that 'no positive conclusion
can be reached.'

"Dr. Harley (*Practitioner*, vol. iii. p. 163) declares that it
does not affect the arteries when applied locally.

"Dr. Fraser, who made 331 experiments with the drug,
chiefly on rabbits, contradicts this, and says he has demonstrated that the local application of the drug *produces dilatation
of the arteries (Wood,* p. 316)."--*The Futility of Experiments
with Drugs on Animals,* by Edward Berdoe (London, 1889)
p. 16.

—— The same.   Macaulay.

JAMES MACAULAY, M.A., M.D., F.R.C.S.Ed., London. (A.V.)

"Calabar bean was reported to be a very dangerous poison,
and Sir Robert Christison determined to try its effect upon
himself—a very ' fair experiment on a living animal ;' as was
that of Sir James Simpson and Dr. Keith in testing the effect
of chloroform as an anæsthetic. Of course, Sir Robert Christison proceeded with extreme caution, and apportioned the dose
with much care, finding the effects such as had been reported
by the missionaries in Africa. He then remitted the further
examination to his assistant, Dr. Fraser, who, in course of
experiments, noticed the remarkable effects of the bean on the
pupil. With due caution, as in Sir Robert Christison's case,
this effect might have been more certainly and directly
observed in the human subject, and with no more danger or
inconvenience than with other poisonous substances which
in minute quantites, are used as medicines. At all events, it
is trifling with the question to single out this physiological
fact as an example of the improvements in medical practice
due to vivisection !"--"*Vivisection*" *Prize Essay* (London,
1881), pp. 49-50.

CAMPHOR, Monobromated.   Berdoe.

EDWARD BERDOE, M.R.C.S., L.R.C.P.Ed., London.   (A.V.)

"Bourneville says, after having performed a number of experiments upon animals with this drug. that it *lowers the temperature, lowers the pulse, and causes sleep.*

"Trasbot experimented with the same drug in a similar manner upon dogs, and found that it *neither lowered the temperature, nor pulse, nor did it cause sleep.*

"Trasbot, in his experiments, says it causes symptoms like those of strychnia.

"Valenti y Vico inferred from his experiments that it was an antidote to strychnia.—(*Stillé, Therapeutics*, 336, 2nd ed.)"— *The Futility of Experiments with Drugs on Animals*, by Edward Berdoe (London, 1889), p. 17.

CANCER GRAFTING.   "Pall Mall Gazette."

"THE PALL MALL GAZETTE," a London Evening Newspaper. (P.V.)

"The sensation created recently in Paris by Professor Cornil's revelations concerning the deliberate grafting of cancerous tumours on living patients is (says the Berlin correspondent of the *Times*) finding a painful counterpart in this country, in consequence of an accusation of similar practices brought by Dr. Eugen Leidig against Dr. Eugen Hahn and Professor von Bergmann. Dr. Hahn has a high reputation as a careful and unusually successful operator, particularly in certain affections of the throat, while the name of Dr. von Bergmann, who fills the chair of surgery at Berlin, has probably been rendered more familiar to English laymen by the prominence which it held in the medical controversies that raged round the death-bed of the late Emperor Frederick. Dr. Leidig declares that Dr. Hahn and Professor von Bergmann have repeatedly experimented on patients in the hospital at Friedrichshain by inoculating them with cancer lymph, adding that the results of these experiments have been published in the medical journals from time to time since the year 1887, and he demands to be informed—first, whether these experiments were conducted with the knowledge and permission of the patients concerned ; secondly, whether the patients were aware that the experiments had no curative purpose ; and, lastly, whether the experiments had the effect of increasing the sufferings of the patients. Dr. Hahn and Professor von Bergmann admit the accuracy of Dr. Leidig's statement, but they say by way of a reply that in every case the patient so operated upon was past recovery. They also affirm that it was necessary for them to select human beings for experiment, inasmuch as none of the lower animals would have been suitable for their purpose. The controversy, so far as it has gone, is anything but reassuring to hospital patients, and has created a widespread feeling of uneasiness in regard to surgical methods which apparently take so little acconnt of human life."—*Pall Mall Gazette*, July 8th, 1891.

CARBOLIC SPRAY.—Lister.—*See* ANTISEPTICS.

CARBONIC ACID GAS.   Berdoe.

EDWARD BERDOE, M.R.C.S., L.R.C.P.Ed., London.   (A.V.)

"The effects of the inhalation of carbonic acid by man do not correspond with those observed in animals. Dogs inhaling this gas in the proportion of one part in nine are thrown into an anæsthetic sleep; but Stillé and Maische say that in similar experiments on man no such anæsthetic influence is pro.!uced. In dogs which have succumbed to a fatal dose, the heart and lungs are found gorged with blood (*Demarquay*). 'In the case of a young man who died in this manner in the Grotto of Pyrmont, the lungs were not engorged, and the heart contained very little blood.—(*Stillé and Maish*, p. 38.)"—*The Futility of Experiments with Drugs on Animals*, by Edward Berdoe (London, 1889), p. 17.

CHLORAL HYDRATE.   Berdoe.

EDWARD BERDOE, M.R.C.S., L.R.C.P.Ed., London.   (A.V.)

"Experimenters with chloral hydrate contradict each other about its physiological action in the most bewildering manner. —(*See* American *Journal of Insanity*, July, 1871, and American *Journal of Medical Science*, April, 1870)."—*The Futility of Experiments with Drugs on Animals* by Edward Berdoe (London, 1889), p. 17.

CHLOROFORM—The Discovery of.   Miller.

JAMES MILLER (The late), Professor in the University of Edinburgh (died 1864).

"The trial proceeded, and the safety as well as suitableness of anæsthesia, by ether, became more and more established. But a new phase was at hand. My friend, Dr. Simpson, had long felt convinced that some anæsthetic agent existed superior to ether, and, in the end of October, 1847, being then engaged in writing a paper on 'Etherization in Surgery,' he began to make experiments on himself and friends in regard to the effects of other respirable matters—other ethers, essential oils, and various gases : chloride of hydro-carbon, acetone, oxide of ethyl, benzine, the vapour of iodoform, etc. The ordinary method of experimenting was as follows :— Each ' operator ' having been supplied with a tumbler, finger glass, saucer, or some such vessel, about a teaspoonful of the respirable substance was put in the bottom of it, and this again was placed in hot water, if the substance happened to be not very volatile. Holding the mouth and nostrils over the vessel's orifice, inhalation was proceeded with, slowly and deliberately, all inhaling at the same time, and each noting the effects as they advanced.

"Most of these experiments were performed after the long day's toil was over, at late night, or early morn ; and when the greater part of mankind was soundly anæsthetized in the arms of common sleep. Late one evening—it was the 4th November, 1847—on returning home after a weary day's labour, Dr. Simpson, with his two friends and assistants, Drs. Keith and Matthews Duncan, sat down to their somewhat hazardous work in Dr. Simpson's dining-room. Having inhaled several substances, but without much effect, it occurred to Dr. Simpson to try a ponderous material, which he had formerly set aside on a lumber table, and which, on account of its great weight, he had hitherto regarded as of no likelihood whatever. That happened to be a small bottle of chloroform. It was searched for, and recovered from beneath a heap of waste paper. And, with each tumbler newly charged, the inhalers resumed their vocation. Immediately an unwonted hilarity seized the party ; they became bright-eyed, very happy, and very loquacious—expatiating on the delicate aroma of the new fluid. The conversation was of unusual intelligence, and quite charmed the listeners—some ladies of the family, and a naval officer, brother-in-law of Dr. Simpson. But suddenly there was a talk of sounds being heard like those of a cotton-mill, louder, and louder, a moment more, then all was quiet, and then—a crash. On awakening, Dr. Simpson's first perception was mental. 'This is far stronger and better than ether,' said he to himself. His second was to note that he was prostrate on the floor, and that among the friends about him there was both confusion and alarm. Hearing a noise, he turned round and saw Dr. Duncan beneath a chair, his jaw dropped, his eyes staring, his head bent half under him, quite unconscious, and snoring in a most determined and alarming manner. More noise still, and much motion ; and then his eyes overtook Dr. Keith's feet and legs, making valorous efforts to overturn the supper-table.

    ✻   ✻   ✻   ✻

" By-and-by, Dr. Simpson having regained his seat, Dr. Duncan having finished his uncomfortable and unrefreshing slumber, and Dr. Keith having come to an arrangement with the table and its contents, the sederunt was resumed. Each expressed himself delighted with this new agent ; and its inhalation was repeated many times that night—one of the ladies gallantly taking her place and turn at the table—until the supply of chloroform was fairly exhausted. In none of these subsequent inhalations, however, was the experiment pushed to unconsciousness. The first event had quite satisfied them of the agent's full power in that way. Afterwards they held their wits entire, and noted the minor effects on themselves and each other. Though the specimen of chloroform was by no means pure, yet they found it much more agreeable and satisfactory in every way than anything else which they had formerly tried; and it required no vote of the party to determine that at length something had been found ' better than ether.' "—*Professor Miller on the " Discovery of Chloroform, : from Principles of Surgery*, pp. 756-758, 2nd Ed. (Edinburgh" Adam and Charles Black ; London : Longmans.)

CHLOROFORM COMMISSION, The Hyderabad.   Brunton.

THOMAS LAUDER BRUNTON, M.D., D.Sc., Lecturer on Materia Medica and Therapeutics, St. Bartholomew's Hospital, London. (V.)

SUMMARY OF EXPERIMENTS.

During the progress of the Hyderabad Commission on chloroform we find 729 experiments noticed in the official report.

Appendix A includes 141 cases, grouped as follows :—

    Series 1.   Dogs chloroformed till death occurred.   8 experiments.

    Series 2.   Artificial respiration tried after large doses of chloroform.   75 experiments.

    Series 3.   Dogs gradually anæsthetized under chloroform (one revived).   17 experiments.

    Series 4.   Dogs rapidly poisoned with large doses of chloroform, no air allowed.   41 experiments.

Among their concluding remarks (*Lancet*, Feb. 22, 1890,

p. 424) we find they decided that : " In no case did cardiac syncope occur ; it is impossible for chloroform vapour to kill a dog by acting primarily upon the heart."

In Appendix C to the report of the Second Commission, there are 588 experiments noted ; in nearly every instance we are told the animal " struggled," or " struggled and resisted as usual " (261). or "yelped loudly" (272). The evident pain inflicted is indicated by the details of many of the experiments. Dogs were put into air-tight cases. wherein the air had previously been saturated with chloroform ; artificial respiration was frequently applied after breathing had stopped, the animals reviving in several cases to become the subjects of new experiments. Doses of phosphorus, injections of strychnine. cocaine, morphine, alcohol. and spirits of ammonia, were administered previously to chloroform being given. In some cases the abdomen was opened before artificial respiration had been applied, as in No. 437, when the dog revived.—*Digest from reports of the Commission, in " The Lancet "* (Feb. 22nd and Mar. 1st, 1890).

CHLOROFORM COMMISSION, The Hyderabad.   Brunton.

THOMAS LAUDER BRUNTON, M.D.Edin., F.R.C.S.Lond., Lecturer on Materia Medica and Therapeutics at St. Bartholomew's Hospital, London. (V.)

" Four hundred and ninety dogs, horses, monkeys, goats, cats, and rabbits used. One hundred and twenty with manometer. All records photographed. Numerous observations on every individual animal. Results most instructive. Danger from chloroform is asphyxia or overdose. None whatever heart direct."—*Telegram from Hyderabad, printed in " Lancet,"* 5th Dec., 1889.

—— The same.   Hewitt.

FREDERICK W. HEWITT, M.D., M.R.C.S., Instructor in and Lecturer on Anæsthetics at the London Hospital, etc. (V.)

" There is much evidence to show that, in whatever way death occurs during chloroform narcosis, the pulse, if carefully watched. usually gives warning of the approach of danger before respiration has become seriously affected. In those cases in which cardiac depression is only indirectly due to the chloroform the initial symptoms are obviously cardiac in origin, and are hence to be detected by alteration in the force and frequency of the pulse. In those cases, too, in which the symptoms are indisputably due to an overdose of chloroform—

such, for example, as the cases reported by the Commission—
the pulse will, in obedience to the fall of vascular tension
(which, as the Commission admits, precedes stoppage of
respiration), give indications of the most important character.
If the Commission could prove that when chloroform is
administered in toxic doses, respiration invariably ceases
whilst the radial pulse is practically unaltered in quality,
we should begin to look upon chloroform as a respiratory
poison only; but these are not the facts, so far as I understand. I cannot avoid the conviction that the Hyderabad
Commission have incurred a grave responsibility in eulogising
chloroform as an anæsthetic for general purposes, and in
recommending administrators to disregard the indications
afforded by the pulse."—*Lancet*, vol. i. 1890, p. 515.

CHLOROFORM COMMISSION, The Hyderabad.   Berdoe.

EDWARD BERDOE, M.R.C.S., L.R.C.P.Ed., London.   (A.V.)

"The dogs of India under the influence of an overdose of
chloroform may die from failure of respiration, and the dogs
of St. Bartholomew's Hospital Laboratory may die from
paralysis of the heart; but I anticipate that very few physicians
or surgeons will modify the practice which prolonged clinical
experience has determined because Dr. Lauder Brunton has
modified his theories at the suggestion of the Chloroform
Commission of a Hindoo Prince. I can imagine circumstances
under which our physiologists would modify every theory in
their books, but fortunately they have as little real influence
on medical practice outside the covers of their works as the
people who conclusively prove that the earth is flat exercise
upon the science of navigation. Naturally a man who has
received a fee of £1,000 to 'discover' something, is strongly
disinclined to say 'ditto' to old theories—even his own—but
when the first excitement has passed away, it will probably be
plainly discerned that what Dr. Brunton has done in regard
to chloroform is simply to have exchanged the London theory
for that of Edinburgh, *i.e.* that the great danger of chloroform
is from arrest of the breathing, and to have 'discovered'—
nothing."—*The Hyderabad Chloroform Commission and Dr.
Lauder Brunton* (London, 1890), pp. 7-8.

—— The same.   Braine.

FRANCIS WOODHOUSE BRAINE, L.R.C.P., F.R.C.S., Lecturer
     on Anæsthetics and Chloroformist, Charing Cross Hospital.   (P.V.)

"Does the Commission prove this?   [The opinion that death

from chloroform is always prefaced by some change or sign of danger in the patient's breathing.] I think not. What it does prove is that in dogs and monkeys and some other animals in India. respiration always gives warning of an overdose, and ceases from one to ten minutes before the heart stops for ever. This is no new statement, for in Snow's work on Anæsthetics, published in 1857, we find the following passage :—' The greater number of experimenters who have killed animals with chloroform have found that the action of the heart continued after the breathing ceased.' . . . A commission reported to the Society of Emulation in Paris, 1855, in all instances in which animals are killed by chloroform. the action of the heart survives the respiration, but they might have administered chloroform to an equal number of human patients without any one of them being cut off by sudden paralysis of the heart. If three cases of death in the human subject are brought forward which have happened in England or in climates resembling ours in which the heart has ceased beating and the patient has gone on breathing afterwards, then I affirm that these cases are of far more importance to us as practical anæsthetists, and far outweigh the 490 experiments which were performed on dogs, monkeys, and other animals in the tropical heat of India."— *From letter on " The Relative Safety of Anæsthetics,"* by Woodhouse Braine, " *Lancet,*" Feb. 8th, 1890.

CHLOROFORM COMMISSION, The Hyderabad.   Braine.

FRANCIS WOODHOUSE BRAINE, L.R.C.P., F.R.C.S., Lecturer on Anæsthetics and Chloroformist, Charing Cross Hospital, London. (P.V.)

" In paragraph 33 of the report, the Committee state that they performed a large number of operations which are reputed to be particularly dangerous from shock, such as extraction of teeth, evulsion of nails, sections of muscles of the eye, etc. These operations were performed in all stages of anæsthesia, and even where the animal was merely stupefied with chloroform ; in no case was there anything suggestive of syncope or failure of the heart's action. And yet in Conclusion VIII. we find ' as a rule, no operation should be commenced until the patient is fully under the influence of the anæsthetic so as to avoid all chance of death from surgical shock or fright.' Now how are we to reconcile these two statements? Is it not apparent that animals do not suffer from surgical shock and cardiac failure, and are in this respect different from human beings? . . . Conclusion IX. states, 'The administrator should be guided as to the effect entirely by the respiration. His only object in producing anæsthesia is to see that the respiration is not interfered with'. From the large experience I have had in administering anæsthetics in England during the last thirty years, I feel absolutely certain that if this deduction is acted upon, the number of fatal cases, even now too numerous. will increase rapidly."—"*The Relative Safety of Anæsthetics*," *a letter in "The Lancet"* (Feb. 8th, 1890), by Woodhouse Braine.

CHLOROFORM COMMISSION, The Hyderabad.   Buxton.

DUDLEY WILMOT BUXTON, M.D., M.R.C.S., Administrator and Lecturer on Anæsthetics, University College and other Hospitals, London. (P.V.)

" Dr. Brunton's work has always been so good, so thorough. and so earnest. that I believe all who are interested in the most important question—Can chloroform be given safely if given properly ?—looked forward with the utmost interest to the feast of reason which he. alike with the other members of the Commission, was to place before us. Now that we have got it, are we happy ? Dispassionate candour compels me to admit that I have been carried no further, although, setting main issues aside, no one can read the suggestive report without gleaning much that is valuable and much that is instructive. In the first place I find no attempt is made to bridge over the great hiatus between experiments on the lower animals and the daily experiments made on man. Possibly this is to come. Again I am disappointed to have no authoritative statements as to whether dogs, monkeys, etc., are liable to syncope under any conditions ; personally, I believe that if they are so, the occurrence must be most rare. Comparing the statements concerning the lower animals with one's own experience, a wide discrepancy occurs ; for every grade of heart weakness finds a record in the note book of every observant anæsthetist, provided his hospital experience is large ; nor can the bulk of such cases be attributed either to primary failure or careless administration."—*Letter to "The Lancet"* (Feb. 15th, 1890) *on the Hyderabad Commission*, by Dudley W. Buxton.

—— The same.   Williams.

WILLIAM ROGER WILLIAMS, F.R.C.S., L.R.C.P., late Hon. Surgeon to the Western General Hospital, London. (P.V.)

" I cannot conclude this letter [on the relative percentage of deaths during the administration of chloroform and ether in St.

Bartholomew's Hospital, 1878–1887 without emphatic protest against the dictum of the Hyderabad Commission, that such deaths must be ascribed entirely to carelessness on the part of the administrators. Such a statement is opposed to all clinical experience, and simply preposterous."—*Letter to* " *The Lancet* " (Feb. 8th, 1890) *on the Relative Safety of Anæsthetics*, by W. Roger Williams.

CHLOROFORM COMMISSION, The Hyderabad.   Silk.

JOHN F. W. SILK, Anæsthetist to Guy's Hospital (Dental School), to the Royal Free Hospital, etc.   (P.V.)

" Next as to the regulations for human administrations which the Commission have drawn up.   They are, to my mind, utterly inconsequent, entirely fallacious.   I cannot possibly admit that any number of experiments on animals ought to outweigh the results of prolonged clinical experience.   As Mr. Braine very aptly remarked, one positive experience should, and does, invalidate a thousand experiments."

* * * * *

" They (the Commission) ask the profession to withhold their judgment until the details of their experiments have been published and fully considered, and express their hopes that if errors have been made, they will be set right *by-and-by*.   At the same time they have not hesitated to draw conclusions from their experiments to give authority for opinions which are confessedly at variance with those usually taught by nearly all practical anæsthetists, and to revert to what I maintain was the erroneous teaching of some forty years ago."—*Letter to* " *The Lancet* " (Feb. 22nd, 1890) *on the Hyderabad Chloroform Commission.*

—— The same.—The Sequel.   Clarke.

JOHN H. CLARKE, M.D., Physician to the Homœopathic Hospital, London.   (A.V.)

" At last, conformably with the Nizam's permission, Surgeon Lieutenant-Colonel Lawrie has arrived ; and according to the *Lancet* of June 2nd, his ' two recently passed men ' have been giving a demonstration of his method of administering chloroform at the London Hospital.   Now, what does this mean ?   It means that, as always happens, the experimenting has been transferred from animals to man—' man,' as usual, meaning ' hospital patient.'   From this it is clear that all the cruel torturings of the myriads of dogs have proved of no avail to settle the question ; to find the action of the drug on man, on man (diseased and healthy) the drug must be tried. Surgeon Lawrie argues for nothing more than Syme laid down without experimenting on animals. He may be right or he may be wrong, or he may be partly both ; be it as it may, it is experience in practice, and not experiments on dogs that will decide, if the question ever is decided. Mr. Treves, who allowed his patients to be chloroformed by Surgeon Lawrie's assistants, is not very enthusiastic of the results."—"*The Hyderabad Chloroform Experiments and their Sequel*," "*Zoophilist*" (London, June, 1894).

CHOLERA—Inoculation against. Haffkine.

J. HAFFKINE, M.D., a Russian by birth, now in India. (V.)

" Inoculation against cholera is being tested on a considerable scale in India by Dr. Haffkine himself, who came to India 18 months ago, and going at once to the cholera infected districts, has, at his own expense, carried out an elaborate series of observations : 32,000 persons have voluntarily submitted themselves to inoculation, and of all these careful records have been kept. The results have varied. Where in a limited and well defined area a certain number of persons have been inoculated and the rest not, the evidence is distinctly in favour of Dr. Haffkine's theory. In some cases the deaths among the inoculated have been eleven times greater than among the non-inoculated, and in others, there were absolutely no cases of cholera among the inoculated. In other cases the results have not been so conclusive. The whole matter is still *sub judice* and in the experimental stage, and no one acknowledges this more freely than Dr. Hafikine himself."—*Report of Indian Medical Congress in " Daily Graphic*," Jan. 24th, 1895.

—— The same—Inoculation against, useless. Metchnikoff.

M. E. METCHNIKOFF, Chef de Service, Pasteur Institute, Paris. (V.)

" In another series of experiments I made some attempts at intestinal vaccination of the human subject, and found that the injection of cholera cultures is not an absolute protection against the pathogenic action of Koch's vibrio. The theory of a condition of unconscious permanent vaccination of persons exempt from cholera has thus been disproved."— *Speech reported in " The Medical Week*," Sept. 27th, 1894.

CHOLERA—Inoculation against, useless. Klein.

EMMANUEL KLEIN, M.D., F.R.S., Lecturer on Anatomy and Physiology, St. Bartholomew's Medical Schools, London. (V.)

" There is absolutely nothing to warrant the assertion that the results produced by the cholera bacillus are comparable to cholera."—*See paper read before the Pathological Society.* " *British Medical Journal,*" March 25th, 1893, p. 632.

" The view of Haffkine and his followers as to the specific nature of the disease induced in the guinea-pig by the intra-peritoneal infection of the cholera bacillus is absolutely untenable.—*Medical Officer's Report to Local Government Board,* 1892-93, p. 377.

—— **The same.**—*See* ACT, THE, EXPERIMENTS UNDER. Klein.

CHOLERA INOCULATIONS. Klein.

EMMANUEL KLEIN, M.D., F.R.S., Lecturer on Anatomy and Physiology, St. Bartholomew's Hospital, London. (V.)

" A few hours (4—8) after the injection the animals show distinct signs of illness ; they become quiet, huddle themselves up in a corner of their cages, and cease to feed ; their tempera-ture is lowered. After about eight to twelve hours this condition is more pronounced; they are now unwilling to walk, and if they attempt this are shaky and unsteady. As a rule the animals are found dead next morning, that is within twenty to twenty-four hours. (p. 370.)

" The *post mortem* examination shows the following appear-ances :—The peritoneum covering the anterior abdominal wall is greatly congested ; this congestion sometimes extends into the abdominal muscles, and is then associated with hæmor-rhages from the minute vessels. The omentum with the serous covering of the intestines is in most cases congested, but in some I have seen the serous coat of the small intestine rather pale ; that of the stomach is, however, always intensely and conspicuously congested. The most pronounced general con-gestion of the peritoneum, associated with hæmorrhage, is noticed in the animals injected with Haffkine's *virus fort.* the peritoneum of the abdominal wall and the muscle itself being of deep purple colour. The serous covering of the liver and the omentum are covered with greyish membranes, sometimes in a thick layer, at other times only a few flakes. The small intestine is either fairly contracted or it is more or less distended by muco-sanguineous contents, which only in a few instances are more or less of a fluid character.

"[Beyond question, therefore, the condition of the small intestine is by no means of a uniform character. It certainly is not of a nature to justify Mr. Hankin (*British Medical Journal*, 1892), when speaking of Haffkine's results, in saying that the condition of the intestine is characteristic of Cholera Asiatica. From my own extensive observations, I should say that if the condition of any organ of such a guinea-pig is indefinite as regards indication of Cholera Asiatica, it is that of the intestine. Moreover, I learn from Mr. Haffkine himself that the above statement of Hankin is not justified by Haffkine's own observations.]" (p. 370.)
— *Extracted from a paper "On the Antagonisms of Microbes," in the Twenty-Second Annual Report of the Local Government Board, 1892-93, Supplement, containing the Report of the Medical Officer for 1892-93.*

CHOLERA—Easy to keep out. Hart.

ERNEST HART, M.R.C.S., Editor *British Medical Journal.* (P.V.)

"There was nothing so easy to keep out and deal with as cholera. The fear of cholera had saved more people than all the epidemics had destroyed and could destroy in fifty years. The knowledge that it is a disease due to dirty water and to filth and uncleanliness had compelled local authorities to take such measures as would prevent the disease. Since 1866, when the quarantine did not keep out cholera, there had been spent in the cities in England £22,000,000 in supplying pure water, and £12,000,000 had been expended on sewage works; now they could snap their fingers at cholera."—*Address at New York: See "British Medical Journal,"* Oct. 28th, 1893, p. 956.

CHOLERA AND FLIES. "Medical Journal."

"THE BRITISH MEDICAL JOURNAL," Organ of the British Medical Association, London. (P.V.)

"Surgeon-Major R. Macrae, in an interesting paper contributed to the *Indian Medical Gazette*, reviews the incidents of the recent outbreak of cholera in the Gaya Gaol from the point of view of the possible conveyance of the contagion from excreta to food through the agency of flies. . . . . No direct proof is tendered of actual conveyance of the cholera poison from stool to food, but the probability of such an occurrence is advanced a stage by the detection by Professor

Haffkine of cholera bacilli in specimens of sterilised milk exposed in new vessels, to which flies were permitted free access in various parts of the gaol. Dr. Macrae contends that even if the comma bacillus be not the cause of cholera, the agency which can disseminate that organism is also competent to distribute any other material which may be the cause."— " British Medical Journal," Dec. 15th, 1894, p. 1388.

See also FLIES AND THE DIFFUSION OF BACTERIA.

CHOLERA, Non-Liability of Animals to.   Koch.
ROBERT KOCH, M.D., Berlin.   (V.)

" As yet we have no certain instance of animals falling spontaneously ill of cholera in periods of cholera. All experiments also. which have hitherto been made on animals with cholera substances, have either given a negative result, or, if they were said to give a positive result, they were not sufficiently supported by evidence, or were disputed by other experimenters. We occupied ourselves, nevertheless, in the most careful and detailed manner. with experiments on animals. Because great value must be laid on the results on white mice obtained by Thiersch, I took fifty mice with me from Berlin, and made all kinds of experiments on them," but " . . . our mice remained healthy. We then made experiments on monkeys, cats. poultry. dogs. and various other animals that we were able to get hold of; but we were never able to arrive at anything in animals similar to the cholera-process. . . . Hence, I think, that all the animals on which we can make experiments, and all those, too, which come into contact with human beings, are not liable to cholera. . . . We must, therefore, dispense with them as a material for affording proofs."— *Koch's* " *Address to the German Board of Health,*" " *British Medical Journal*," Sept. 6th, 1884, page 454.

CHRYSOPHANIC ACID, Contradictory   Berdoe.
   Experiments with.
EDWARD BERDOE, M.R.C.S., L.R.C.P.Ed., London.   (A.V.)

" Experimenters with this drug do not agree respecting its action. Some declare that it is a purgative, while the greater number assure us that it has no such property. They are equally divided as to the question of its elimination from the system after its exhibition.—(*Stillé and Maisch.* p. 42)."—*The Futility of Experiments with Drugs on Animals*, by Edward Berdoe (London, 1889), p. 17.

CITRIC ACID. Berdoe.

EDWARD BERDOE, M.R.C.S., L.R.C.P.Ed., London. (A.V.)

"This acid is prepared from lemon juice. Physiologists have experimented with it upon cats, rabbits, and other animals, with results which should teach medical men how fallacious it is to expect the lower animals to illustrate the uses of medicines proposed to be exhibited on human beings. Citric acid proves to be a powerful poison to these animals; it causes in them the most violent tetanic spasms. In man, however, no spasmodic or any other alarming symptom ever arises from its use (*Stillé and Maisch*, p. 44)."—*The Futility of Experiments with Drugs on Animals*, by Edward Berdoe (London, 1889), pp. 17, 18.

CLAIMS, The Inordinate, for Vivisection. Macaulay.

JAMES MACAULAY, M.A., M.D., F.R.C.S.Ed., London. (A.V.)

"An article (in the *British Medical Journal*, Jan. 9th, 1875, p. 56) concludes with the following sentences, the mere quotation of which will suffice to show the inordinate claims and pretensions of vivisection:—" To record all the facts given to physiology by experiments on animals would simply be to write the history of the science. Therapeutics is yet in its infancy; but *nearly all the facts definitely known regarding the actions of remedies have been gained by experiments on animals* (!) To stop experiments on animals would as surely arrest the progress of physiology, pathology and therapeutics, as an edict preventing the chemist from the use of the retort, test-tube, acids and alkalies, would arrest the progress of chemistry.' On reading this, I wondered what would be the effect of such an assertion in the minds of the intelligent readers of the *British Medical Journal*—of those, at least, outside the circles of vivisectors, and their advocates or apologists. Have all the observations of clinical medicine, of pathological anatomy, of pathological histology, and pathological chemistry been vain and fruitless? Have all the labours recorded in books of medicine and surgery, in medical reports and the transactions of societies, in practical manuals and text-books, and in our official pharmacopœias and dispensatories, been delusive and misleading? Almost the whole classic literature of the profession belongs to a time when, in England, the practice of vivisection was comparatively unknown, and when its results were regarded with doubt, if not with condemnation. Have all the generalizations and conclusions of past experience been superseded by the results of this new method of research ? Has the healing art, in short, been wholly revolutionized since vivisectors came into the field ? The official reports of the Registrar-General, the pages of our medical journals, the case-books of our practitioners, refute the claim. Till some better statement can be given of ' what vivisection has done for humanity,' respectable medical men will keep to the old paths—paths of honour, and not of shame."— *Vivisection, A Prize Essay*, by James Macaulay (London, 1881), p. 51.

CLINICAL AND EXPERIMENTAL METHODS. — *See* DANGERS OF THE EXPERIMENTAL METHOD.

CLINICAL AND PATHOLOGICAL STUDY, Macaulay. the True Source of Knowledge.

JAMES MACAULAY, M.A., M.D., F.R.C.S. Ed., London. (A.V.)

" If physiology owes much to comparative anatomy, and also to physics, and to chemistry, it owes much to pathology. Along with pathology is included morbid anatomy, or the *post mortem* inspection of structure, for investigation of the results of diseased action in life. When the writer was a student at the University of Edinburgh, there was a good deal of discussion about vivisection, then attracting considerable notice, from the experiments of Majendie and other French physiologists. He well remembers Dr. Abercrombie's strongly expressed opinion about such experiments, and his advice to depend on clinical and pathological study for the knowledge that could be applied in the practice of medicine. Having had his attention thus early directed to the claims of experiment, as compared with observation, he has ever since watched the progress of vivisection ; and a review of the results now, after forty years, confirms the belief that Dr. Abercrombie's opinion and advice were right. And certainly not the least injurious influence of the present rage for experimenting is its tendency to withdraw attention from seeking the advancement of physiology, as well as medicine, through clinical and pathological study."—*Vivisection, A Prize Essay*, by James Macaulay (London, 1881), pp. 53, 54.

COCCULUS INDICUS, Varying Effects Berdoe. of, on Men and Animals.

EDWARD BERDOE, M.R.C.S., L.R.C.P.Ed., London. (A.V.)

" Cocculus Indicus is a well-known poison used for catching
G

fish by intoxicating them ; under its influence they whirl round, and lie motionless on the water.   In dogs and other animals it causes muscular tremors, convulsions, and tetanic spasms.   It is remarkable that there is no case on record where such effects have been produced on man by this drug.   We have cases of stomach irritation, congestion of the brain and death, but no spasmodic phenomena.—(*Stillé Therapeutics*, 2nd Ed., p. 436),"
—*The Futility of Experiments with Drugs on Animals*, by Edward Berdoe (London, 1889), p. 18.

COMMISSION, THE ROYAL, expressed no Opinion as to the Abuses of Vivisection.   Hutton.

RICHARD HOLT HUTTON, Editor of the *Spectator*, and a Member of the Royal Commission of 1875.   (R.)

" ' F.R.S.' has absolutely no right to say in his letter to *The Times* of yesterday that 'the Royal Commission of 1876 on subjecting live animals to experiment for scientific purposes, which was presided over by Lord Cardwell, and included such a declared opponent of vivisection as Mr. Hutton, failed, after receiving evidence from all quarters, to bring to light a single instance of wanton cruelty or any serious abuse in this country.' Lord Cardwell never proposed to us to pass any opinion on the extent to which abuses had or had not been exposed. The report expressly states :—'We have not thought it our duty, the majority of us not having had professional training, to decide upon matters of differing professional opinion, but we have been much struck by the consideration that severe experiments have been engaged in for the purpose of establishing results which have been considered inadequate to justify that severity by persons of very competent authority.' (*Report*, p. 17.) Notoriously, the Commission could not have agreed in any unanimous report had it been proposed to declare that no abuses had been brought to light. . . . It should, however, be known that it certainly was not the testimony of the Royal Commissioners that no abuses had been brought to light ; and we all concurred in saying :—' Besides the cases in which inhumanity exists, we are satisfied that there are others in which carelessness and indifference prevail to an extent sufficient to form a ground for legislative interference.' (*Report*, p. 17.) That is not in any sense a whitewashing judgment."—*Letter in* " *The Times*," by R. H. Hutton, Jan. 13, 1885.

CONSUMPTION.—*See* TUBERCULOSIS.

COPPER, SULPHATE OF, Cruel Experiments with, on Animals.

Berdoe.

EDWARD BERDOE, M.R.C.S., L.R.C.P.Ed., London. (A.V.)

" Atrociously cruel experiments upon dogs have been tried with this poison. Given by the mouth it excites violent vomiting, but some physiologists, to prevent this, have tied the gullet, and thereby have caused convulsions and paralysis. Yet Levi and Barduzzi gave a horse daily 15 grains of sulphate of copper for 30 days without injury. An ass was subjected to the same treatment with similar results."—*The Futility of Experiments with Drugs on Animals*, by Edward Berdoe (London, 1889), p. 18.

CORROSIVE SUBLIMATE (Perchloride of Mercury), Contradictions of Experiments with.

Berdoe.

EDWARD BERDOE, M.R.C.S., L.R.C.P.Ed., London. (A.V.)

" Drs. Wright and Wilbouchewitch (*Archiv de Phys.*, Sept., 1874) experimented with corrosive sublimate upon rabbits, and found that it *very greatly diminished* the number of the red blood corpuscles.

" Dr. Keyes (Amer. *Jour. Med. Sci.*, Jan., 1876) did the same, and he says that it *increases* the number of the red blood corpuscles."—*The Futility of Experiments with Drugs on Animals*, by Edward Berdoe (London, 1889), p. 19.

CROTON OIL, Contradictory Effects of, on Animals and Man.

Berdoe.

EDWARD BERDOE, M.C.R.S., L.R.C.P.Ed., London. (A.V.)

" Armand Moreau experimented with the intestines of living dogs by cutting them open and putting croton oil into them, and obtained opposite results to those obtained by M. Thivey, who did the same."—(*Gaz. Med.*, 1871.)

" Hertwig and Bucheim (*Virchow's Archiv*, xii. 1) injected croton oil into the veins of animals, and found that *purgation did not follow*.

" Conwell did exactly the same, but with a *contrary result*. Stillé (*Therap.*, vol. ii. p. 451) says that it will sometimes purge human beings even when applied externally."—*The Futility of Experiments with Drugs on Animals*, by Edward Berdoe (London, 1889), p. 19.

CRUEL EXPERIMENTS under Curare.   Sanderson.

JOHN BURDON SANDERSON, M.D., F.R.S., Regius Professor of Medicine, University of Oxford. (V.)

" In 1863 the lamented v. Bezold published his well-known researches on the nervous system of the heart. Among a number of other less important discoveries, he showed for the first time the nature and extent of the influence exercised by the brain and spinal cord on the circulation of the blood. He found that when, in a curarised rabbit or dog, the spinal cord is severed from the brain, the arterial pressure sinks very considerably, while at the same time the number and extent of the contractions of the heart are diminished ; and that if, on the other hand, the upper end of the divided spinal cord is irritated below the point of section, the arterial pressure rises to its original level and the heart to its previous activity.

" The leading experiment is as follows ;—Two centigrammes of curare, dissolved in a cubic centimetre of water, are injected below the skin, and immediately after artificial respiration is begun. This dose is sufficient, as was first shown by v. Bezold himself, to paralyse the extremities so completely that neither stimulation of the cord nor of any muscular nerve produces the slightest contraction of voluntary muscles, while, as we shall see on another occasion, it is not sufficient to interfere with the action of the heart. Respiration of course ceases. but it is maintained, as I have said, mechanically. the means employed for the purpose being a pair of bellows the tube of which communicates with a cannula adapted to the trachea of the animal.

" The membrane between the atlas and the occipital bone having been previously exposed and one of the carotid arteries connected with the manometer of the kymograph, observations are taken of the arterial pressure and of the frequency of the pulse. This done, the spinal cord is divided at the atlas. Immediately the rate of pulsation is diminished, say from 140 to 100, and after a few seconds the arterial pressure sinks, say from three or four inches to one or two. Needles are then inserted into the spinal cord, one at the upper edge of the axis, both of which are connected with the secondary coil of Dubois' induction apparatus. At once the heart beats more frequently and vigorously and the mercurial column attains its former level.

" The next step in the experiment is the destruction of the cerebro-spinal cardiac nerves. These nerves, as you know, reach the heart or leave it either through the vagi or the sympathetic.

" The destruction of the nerves is best effected with the galvanic cautery, the action of which is more certain and more easily controlled than any other agent which could be employed. It answers the purpose so completely that in careful subsequent dissection it is found that every nerve is served. As soon as the destruction of the nerves is effected the spinal cord is again excited, great care being taken that the strength of the current shall be the same as in the previous observation.

" There are, however, in these and other respects considerable differences in the results observed in different animals the conditions of which have not yet been determined.

" Upon another dog, under partial anæsthesia, he divided with a fine curved scalpel the corpus striatum and optic thalamus on one side, the corpus callosum having previously been cut through. The electrodes were then placed on the convolutions above and behind the sylvian fissure. Contraction resulted, when the current was strong, not only in the fore leg of the opposite side, but also in the hind leg. In another experiment he removed the whole cerebral masses above the varolii, and applied the electrodes to the surface of the section. Muscular contractions resulted, limited to the fore limbs, right and left."—*Lecture at Univ. Coll., London, in The Lancet*, No. 2630, p. 136. (*Blue Book, Roy. Com.*, London, 1876, *Appendix* iv., pp. 380, 381.)

CRUEL EXPERIMENTS. Boy and Dog United. "Standard."

"THE STANDARD," London Daily Newspaper (Evening Edition), Feb. 7th, 1891. (P.V.)

" Our readers will remember a disgusting story of the attempt by a New York doctor to graft the bone of a dog on the leg of a boy. Here is the conclusion from the *Evening Standard*, February 7th :—' With regard, however, to the bone-grafting experiment, in which the bones of a dog were used, the surgeons declare it to be a complete failure. The little boy has, it is stated, undergone no fewer than six operations, but the bones of the dog cannot be brought to unite with his. A temporary union, it seems, was effected, which did not last, and could not last, in the opinion of medical men, without the infusion of the dog's blood—an indispensable factor to the permanent knitting of the bones together. Of course, it was not possible to resort to such an expedient, and all that could be done was to declare the operation a failure. The question, as it is remarked, not unnaturally suggests itself whether the poor child ought to have been tortured as he has been since the first operation in November last, and to have had severe suffering inflicted on him for the sake of scientific experiment.' We are delighted to find a British newspaper taking this view. We hope to hear more of it."—*The Zoophilist* (London), March 2nd, 1891, p. 206.

CRUELTIES OF THE FARMYARD.—*See* FARMYARD CRUELTIES.

CRUELTY OF VIVISECTION.   Bell.

BELL, SIR CHARLES (the late), M.E.C.S., 1797 ; M.R.C.S., 1812 ; Lecturer on Physiology, University College, London, 1826 ; Professor of Surgery, University of Edinburgh, 1831 (born 1778 ; died 1842). (V.)

" After delaying long on account of the unpleasant nature of the operation, I opened the spinal canal of a rabbit, and cut the posterior roots of the nerves of the lower extremity—the creature still crawled—but I was deterred from repeating the experiment by the protracted cruelty of the dissection. I reflected that the experiment would be satisfactory if done on an animal recently knocked down and insensible—that whilst I experimented on a living animal there might be a trembling or action excited in the muscles by touching a sensitive nerve, which motion it would be difficult to distinguish from that produced more immediately through the influence of the motor nerves."— *Nervous System of the Human Body* (Longman & Co., 1830), p. 31.

—— The same. "No Case of Wanton   Colam. Cruelty" Explained.

JOHN COLAM, Secretary to the Royal Society for the Prevention of Cruelty to Animals. (R.)

" You would treat cases of wilful cruelty, if they exist at all in this country, as exceptional cases rather than as fairly chargeable upon any want of proper sentiment on the part of the profession ?—Undoubtedly with regard to wanton cruelty. I do not know that I know of a single case of wanton cruelty, by which I mean suffering caused without any object except to gratify a cruel mind.

　　　*　　　　*　　　　*　　　　*　　　　*

" But you think that experiments are performed which are in

their nature beyond any legitimate province of science, and
that the pain which they inflict, is pain which is not justifiable
to inflict, even for the scientific object which they have in view?
—That is the opinion of our society."—*Evid. Roy. Com.* (London, 1876), Q. 1546 and 1549.

CRUELTY OF VIVISECTION, Beyond Question. Borel.

F. BOREL, M.D., Ex-Chief of a Hospital (V).

" Permit a vivisector, past and present, and future, if it were
necessary for the good of science and mankind to tell those good
people who believe seriously that the animals experimented on
by M. Pasteur do not suffer, that they are deceiving themselves ; my personal experience of fifteen years' practice gives
me the right formally to deny the truth of that. I have vivisected birds, horses, frogs, rabbits, monkeys, and above all,
dogs ; and I can affirm three things :—

" 1. That it is nearly completely impossible to employ
anæsthetics upon them so as to render them insensible ; as,
for example, ether, chloroform, chloral, opium (morphine.
codeine). canabis indica (haschich), etc.

" 2. That the sufferings of the animals are so great after
the experiments that they are altogether stupefied ; the most
ferocious dogs allow themselves to be used, later on, with
the indifference of sheep : one must not absolutely confound
their tranquillity with the relief given to a man after a
necessary surgical operation, but as the apathy and indifference
of a martyr. I have experimented on mad dogs ; the second
time I placed them on the table they were as gentle as rabbits.
For the rest, it may be said in passing, mad dogs are already
so ill that in general they are very gentle.

" 3. The employment of curare, far from diminishing
sensibility, augments it exceedingly ; more than that, the use
of it necessitates tracheotomy beforehand, to make them
respire artificially, because the curare totally paralyzes all
voluntary movements, and thus they would otherwise suffocate.

" Any one who is accustomed to a laboratory, to physiology,
or to pathological experiments knows that animals suffer when
vivisected, and greatly, until death comes to deliver them.
No ! It is necessary for M. Pasteur to have living animals to
support his thesis : this letter is not the place to inquire
whether he is right or wrong ; but that I maintain, I,
pathologist and lately chief of a hospital, that he has imposed
upon brave men whose confidence he has won, when he
pretends that these animals do not suffer. To listen to him,

one would say they come voluntarily to submit themselves to experiments, to procure pleasures hitherto unknown."—*Letter in the "Pall Mall Gazette,"* Aug. 5th, 1889.

CRUELTY AND HORROR OF VIVISECTION.   Guinness.

ARTHUR GUINNESS, M.D., F.R.C.S.I., Cheltenham.   (A.V.)

" When I reflect on the abominable cruelties inflicted on animals by such callous beings as M. de Cyon, and many others (I regret to say) of my own countrymen, I can truly say a thrill of horror comes over me, and also disgust, when I think that mankind can be so degraded as to commit such horrors. It behoves, then, every man. more especially medical men, to come forward and denounce it firmly and boldly. and by all means in their power to endeavour to get the Bill passed for its total prohibition."—*Letter in the "Oxford and Cambridge Undergraduates' Journal,"* Oct. 23rd, 1884.

—— The same.   Majendie and his victim.   Leffingwell.

ALBERT LEFFINGWELL, M.D., Cambridge Mass., U.S.A.   (R.)

" There is a certain experiment—one of the most excruciating that can be performed—which consists in exposing the spinal cord of the dog for the purpose of demonstrating the functions of the spinal nerves.   It is one, by the way, which Dr. Wilder forgot to enumerate in his summary of the 'four kinds of experiments,' since it is not the 'cutting operation' which forms its chief peculiarity or to which special objection would be made.   At present all this preliminary process is generally performed under anæsthetics; it is an hour or two later, when the animal has partly recovered from the severe shock of the operation, that the wound is reopened and the experiment begins.   It was during a class-demonstration of this kind by Majendie, before the introduction of ether, that the circumstance occurred which one hesitates to think possible in a person retaining a single spark of humanity or pity.   ' I recall to mind,' says Dr. Latour, who was present at the time, ' a poor dog, the roots of whose vertebral nerves Majendie desired to lay bare, to demonstrate Bell's theory, which he claimed as his own.   The dog, mutilated and bleeding, twice escaped from under the implacable knife, and threw its front paws around Majendie's neck, licking as if to soften his murderer and ask for mercy ! I confess I was unable to endure that heart-rending spectacle.'   It was probably in reference to this experiment that Sir Charles Bell, the greatest English physiologist of our century, writing to his brother in 1822, informs him that he hesitates to go on with his investigations. ' You may think me silly,' he adds, ' but I cannot perfectly convince myself that I am authorized in nature or religion to do these cruelties.' "—" *Vivisection,*" *Lippincott's Magazine*, Aug., 1884, p. 129.

CRUELTY OF VIVISECTORS.   Bernard.

CLAUDE BERNARD (the late), M.D., Paris, 1843 ; Pupil and Assistant to M. Majendie ; Prof. of Medicine at Faculty of Science, Paris ; Member of the Academy of Science ; succeeded Majendie as Professor of Experimental Physiology at the College of France in 1855 ; Prof. Gen. Physiol. at Museum, 1868. (Born 1813 ; died 1878.) (V.)

" A physiologist is no ordinary man. He is a learned man, a man possessed and absorbed by a scientific idea. He does not hear the animals' cries of pain. He is blind to the blood that flows. He sees nothing but his idea, and organisms which conceal from him the secrets he is resolved to discover."— *Introd. à l'Etude de la Médecine Expérimentale* (Paris, 1855), p. 180.

—— The same.   Cyon.

ELIAS DE CYON, Professor of Physiology at St. Petersburg. (V.)

" The true vivisector must approach a difficult vivisection with joyful excitement. . . . He who shrinks from cutting into a living animal, he who approaches a vivisection as a disagreeable necessity, may be able to repeat one or two vivisections, but he will never be an artist in vivisection. . . . The sensation of the physiologist when, from a gruesome wound, full of blood and mangled tissue, he draws forth some delicate nerve thread . . . has much in common with that of a sculptor."—*Methodik,* p. 15.

—— The same.   Cheyne.

WILLIAM WATSON CHEYNE, M.B.Edin., F.R.C.S.Eng., Professor of Surgery, King's College ; Surgeon, King's College Hospital, London. (V.)

" I took a mixture of equal parts of croton oil and olive oil, sterilized it, introduced it into sterilized glass capsules, which were then sealed at both ends. An incision was made antiseptically in the muscles of the back of a rabbit, and the tube introduced into the muscles ; the wound was then stitched with catgut, and an antiseptic dressing applied. The result was that in a certain number of cases the wound healed by first intention, and the glass capsule remained embedded in the muscles as an unirritating foreign body. After a certain time had elapsed the capsule was broken by slight pressure against the spine, and thus the croton oil was brought into contact with the tissues. In one experiment performed in this way the capsule was broken fifty-four days after its insertion, and the animal was killed twenty-seven days later."—*The British Medical Journal* (Feb. 25th, 1888), p. 409.

CRUELTY OF VIVISECTORS.   Brachet.

JEAN LOUIS BRACHET (b. 1789; d. at Lyons, 1858), Professor of Physiology, School of Medicine, Paris. (V.)

"Dr. Brachet says, 'I inspired a dog with the greatest aversion for me by plaguing and inflicting some pain or other upon it, as often as I saw it; when this feeling was carried to its height, so that the animal became furious as soon as it saw or heard me, I put out its eyes. I could then appear before it without its manifesting any aversion. I spoke, and immediately its barkings and furious movements proved the passion which animated it. I destroyed the drum of its ears, and disorganized the internal ear as much as I could; and when an intense inflammation which was excited had rendered it deaf, I filled up its ears with wax. It could no longer hear at all. Then I went to its side, spoke aloud and even caressed it, without its falling into a rage,—it seemed even sensible of my caresses.' Dr. Brachet repeated the same experiment on another dog, and assures us that the result was the same."— *From " Vivisections and Painful Experiments on Living Animals,"* by Gimson Gimson, M.D., M.R.C.S. (London, 1879), p. 143.

—— The same.   Majendie.

FRANCOIS MAJENDIE, M.D., Member of the Academies of Sciences and of Medicine (born 1783; died 1855). (V.)

"Dr. Majendie says, 'It is droll to see animals skip and jump about of their own accord, after you have taken out all their brains a little before the optic tubercles;' and as to 'new-born kittens,' he says, 'they tumble over in all directions, and walk so nimbly, if you cut out their hemispheres, that it is quite astonishing."—*Journal de Physiologie*, t. iii. p. 155.

CRUELTY OF VIVISECTORS. Klein.

EMMANUEL KLEIN, M.D., F.R.S., Lecturer on Anatomy and
Physiology at the Medical School of St. Bartholomew's. (V.)

"*Chairman :* What is your own practice with regard to the
use of anæsthetics in experiments that are otherwise painful ?
Dr. Klein : Except for teaching purposes, for demonstration,
I never use anæsthetics where it is not necessary for convenience. If I demonstrate, I use anæsthetics. If I do experiments for my inquiries in pathological research, except for
convenience sake, as for instance on dogs and cats, I do not
use them. On frogs and the lower animals I never use them.
When you say that you only use them for convenience sake, do
you mean that you have no regard at all to the sufferings of
the animals ?—No regard at all. You are prepared to establish
that as a principle which you approve ?—I think that with regard to an experimenter, a man who conducts special research.
and performs an experiment, he has no time, so to speak, for
thinking what will the animal feel or suffer. His only purpose
is to perform the experiment, to learn as much from it as
possible, and to do it as quickly as possible. Then for your
own purposes you disregard entirely the question of the suffering of the animal in performing a painful experiment ?—I do.
Why do you regard it then when it is for a demonstration ?
—Because I know that there is a great deal of feeling against it
in this country, and when it is not necessary, one should not
perhaps act against the opinion or the belief of certain individuals of the auditorium. One must take regard of the feelings and opinions of those people before whom one does the
experiment. Then am I wrong in attributing to you that you
separate yourself entirely from the feeling which you observe
to prevail in this country in regard to humanity to animals ?—
I separate myself as an investigator from myself as a teacher.
But in regard to your proceedings as an investigator, you are
prepared to acknowledge that you hold as entirely indifferent
the sufferings of the animal which is subjected to your investigation ?—Yes. Do you believe that that is a general practice
on the Continent, to disregard altogether the feelings of the
animals ?—I believe so. But you believe that, generally speaking, there is a very different feeling in England ?—Not among
the physiologists ; I do not think there is."—*Minutes of Evidence Royal Commission* (London, 1876), Q. 6538 to 6550.

—- **The same.** Martin.

H. NEWELL MARTIN, Professor of Biology, Johns Hopkins
University, Baltimore, U.S.A. (V.)

" After dividing the skin in the middle line, I have always

removed a piece of the skull with a small trephine applied in a lozenge-shaped area which is seen to be bounded on the sides by four small vessels. The posterior edge of the opening thus made extends back to about opposite the posterior margin of the cerebral hemispheres, and the aperture was enlarged with scissors until the front edges of the optic lobes came into view. These were carefully and completely separated by a cataract knife from the parts of the brain in front of them, and the latter were removed from the cranial cavity; the incision in the skull being usually carried forwards to facilitate this removal. The edges of the skin were then brought carefully in contact, without sutures. and the animal placed in a dish containing a little water and left until the wound healed up. . . . They [frogs] were not fed. as experience showed me that for the week or two during which I desired to keep them, they did better without food ; or at least without the exhausting struggle which the attempt to open their mouths called forth."—*Journal of Physiology*, vol. i. p. 155.

CRUELTY OF VIVISECTORS. Bradford.

J. ROSE BRADFORD, D.Sc., M.R.C.S., Assistant Professor of Clinical Medicine, University College, London. (V.)

In a paper on " The effects of the destruction of the tympanic plexus in the dog," the details of which are exceedingly cruel, it is narrated that a muscle known as the digastric was dissected out and turned aside "in the usual manner," so as to expose the " tympanic bulla," " it was then trephined and the opening enlarged with bone forceps ; the interior of the tympanum (or middle ear) was next scraped out with a small sharp Volckman's spoon, and then the cavity was scrubbed out with a solution of chloride of zinc; *this, as is well known from surgical practice, destroys everything it comes in contact with.* The animals were killed thirty-eight and twenty days after the operation."—*Condensed from " The Journal of Physiology,"* vol. ix. p. 309, etc.

—— The same. Hoggan.

GEORGE HOGGAN. M.B. (the late), a witness before the Royal Commission, 1875 (born 1837 ; died 1891). (R.)

" Paul Bert's experiment on a curarized dog was of the following nature : The side of the face, the side of the neck, the side of the foreleg, interior of the belly, and the hip were dissected out in order to lay bare, respectively, the sciatic, etc., nerves.

These were excited by electricity for ten consecutive hours."—
Evid. Roy. Com. (London, 1876), Q. 4111, *and* "*Archives de Physiologie*," vol. ii. 1869, p. 650.

CRUELTY OF VIVISECTORS.—See also " WANTON EXPERIMENTS " and " PROLONGED PAIN."

CURARE. • Bernard.

CLAUDE BERNARD (the late), M.D., Pupil and Assistant of Majendie : Professor of Experimental Physiology, Collège de France, Paris (born 1813 ; died 1878). (V.)

"Curare acting on the nervous system only suppresses the action of the motor nerves, leaving sensation intact. Curare is not an anæsthetic.

※　　※　　　　　※　　※

"Curare renders all movement impossible. but it does not hinder the animal from suffering, and from being conscious of pain."—*Revue Scientifique*, 1871-2, p. 892 ; also vol. vi. p. 591.
" Thus all their descriptions offer us a pleasant and tranquil picture of death by curare. A gentle sleep seems to occupy the transition from life to death. But it is nothing of the sort : the external appearances are deceitful.

※　　※　　※　　※

" In this motionless body, behind that glazing eye,and with all the appearance of death, sensitiveness and intelligence persist in their entirety. The corpse before us hears and distinguishes all that is done around it. It suffers when pinched or irritated ; in a word, it has still consciousness and volition, but it has lost the instruments which serve to manifest them."—*Revue des deux Mondes*, vol. 53, second series (Sept. 1st, 1864), pp. 173 and 182.

CURARE, The Effects of. Holmgren.

F. HOLMGREN, Professor of Physiology, Upsala University. (V.)

" There is a poison (curare) which lames every spontaneous movement, leaving all other functions untouched. This venom is therefore the most cruel of all poisons. It changes us instantly into a living corpse, which hears and sees and knows everything, but is unable to move a single muscle, and under its influence no creature can give the faintest indication of its hopeless condition. The heart alone continues to beat."—*Holmgren's " Physiology of Present Times*," 1868, p. 231.

CURARE. Bernard.

CLAUDE BERNARD (the late), Pupil and Assistant of Majendie Professor of Experimental Physiology, Collège de France, Paris (born 1813 ; died 1878). (V.)

" Curare is now employed in a vast number of experiments as a means of restraining the animals. There are but few observations of which the narrative does not commence by notifying that they were made on a curarized dog."—*Physiologie Opératoire* (Paris, 1879), p. 168.

—— The same. Schiff.

MORITZ SCHIFF, M.D., Professor of Physiology at Geneva. (V.)

" It is nothing but hypocrisy to wish to impose on oneself or on others the belief that the curarized animal does not always feel pain."—*Sopra il Metodo seguito negli esperimenti sugli animali Viventi, etc.*, p. 37.* (*Firenze, Andrea Bettini.*)

—— Utility of. Sharpey.

WILLIAM SHARPEY (the late), M.D.Elin., 1823 ; LL.D.Edin. ; F.R.C.S.Edin., 1830 ; F.R.S., F.R.S.E. ; Prof. Anat. and Physiol. Univ. of London, 1836 (born 1802 ; died 1881). (V.)

" The chief use of employing curare is to render the animal

---

* In the second edition of this pamphlet, Dr. Schiff writes (before the above sentence) as follows, pp. 34, 35, 36 :—

" In the first edition of this little work, we could not speak of curare because we could not consider it as an anæsthetic. Since that time we have made new experiments on frogs, and found that curare given in *great doses* really abolishes sensibility, but that it only acts as an anæsthetic a long time after having destroyed voluntary movements and automatic respiration. Among mammals it is impossible to make such experiments as should indicate exactly when sensation ceases after the beginning of the poisoning. But it is certain that even here sensibility still exists when every voluntary movement has ceased, and we have no right to assume that a mammal poisoned with curare is insensible because it cannot manifest its sensibility with ordinary movements and cries. In that condition we must admit that the persistency of consciousness and of pain is possible during all the time in which an animal still responds to a strong impression, either by a manifest contraction of the veins or of the softer involuntary muscles, which contractions we cannot discern directly but only through the complicated methods afforded by science. If we should wait to experiment on the curarized animal till after the cessation of all these movements, then the experiment would have no purpose or value, because the experiments are generally made expressly to reveal these movements," p. 36.

quite still; that is the great purpose of it. What Mr. Hutton says is quite true, that it is not generally recognised as an anæsthetic, and therefore not used as an anæsthetic.—Then it is a contrivance to save to the operator the trouble which the manifestation of pain by the animal might occasion him ? It facilitates the operation at any rate."—*Evid. Roy.Com.* (London, 1876), Q. 462, 3.

CURARE, Used to render Animals passive. Brunton.

THOMAS LAUDER BRUNTON, M.D., D.Sc., Lecturer on Materia Medica and Therapeutics at St. Bartholomew's Hospital, London. (V.)

" Then the purpose for which wourali [curare] is used is in order to keep the animal quiet, to make the experiment an easier one to conduct ?—Yes, in frogs and in the higher animals it is to get rid of some of the effects which might be due to irritation of the nerve centres. For example, this is the case in some physiological experiments that have been made in Germany by irritation of various parts of the nervous system of the upper part of the spinal cord [*i.e.* medulla]. You want to ascertain the influence of that part upon the vascular system generally, the system of blood-vessels, and you want to ascertain that alone. If you irritate the upper part of the cord after you have given wourali, you only get the action upon the blood-vessels ; but if you were to irritate this part without giving wourali previously, you would get the irritation conducted all down the ordinary motor nerves, and get all the muscles set into violent action ; the action of the muscles would react upon the vessels, and you would get the whole experiment disturbed."—*Evid. Roy. Com.* (London, 1876), Q. 5,742.

—— The same. Its Paralysing Effect. Liouville.

HENRI LIOUVILLE (the late), M.D., Paris, Chief Director of the Laboratory, Hotel Dieu. (V.)

" Liouville gives a description of a case where an overdose had been given, and artificial respiration had to be kept up till the patient recovered. He says, ' The patient then related all he had felt, the preservation of the intellect, the annihilation of all power of movement, of which he gave a clear account, witnessing all that went on around him, without being able to take any part in it, the fears freely expressed by some young assistants present being by no means reassuring to him.' "—*Bulletin Général Thérapeutique*, Nov., 1865, p. 404.

CURE OF DISEASE—Experiments not directed to the.

Richet.

CHARLES RICHET, M.D., Professor of Physiology, Faculty of Medicine, Paris. (V.)

" I do not believe that a single experimenter says to himself when he gives curare to a rabbit, or cuts the spinal marrow of a dog, or poisons a frog : ' Here is an experiment which will relieve or will cure the disease of some men.' No. in truth, he does not think of that ! He says to himself, ' I will clear up an obscure point, I will seek out a new fact.' And this scientific curiosity, which alone animates him, is explained by the high idea he has formed of Science. This is why we pass our days in fœtid laboratories (*dans les salles nauséabondes*), surrounded by groaning creatures, in the midst of blood and suffering, bent over palpitating entrails."—*Revue des deux Mondes*, Feb. 15th, 1883.

DANGERS OF THE EXPERIMENTAL METHOD.

Clark.

SIR ANDREW CLARK, Bart. (the late), M.D.Aberd., F.R.C.P., etc. (born 1839 : died 1893.) (P.V.)

" For whatever purpose they may be employed : however carefully they may be designed and executed : however successful may be the precaution taken to exclude error, experiments have their subtle difficulties and dangers, which are perilous to truth and cannot be wholly averted. By the prestige of precision, which often undeservedly they possess, undue weight is attached to their results ; and by the assumption that in like conditions the results would be the same in man as in the lower animals, flagrant errors are committed, and currency is given to false or inadequate generalisations. The experimenter interprets the results of his experiments by the light of their structural results ; he forgets, or he ignores, the life history of the processes by which they have been evolved, and he takes no account of the fact, beyond controversy, that different clinical states find occasionally the same structural expression. In such circumstances doubt is inevitable, and it is only to clinical medicine that any just appeal for its solution can be made. To her, at last, all such experiments must be brought for trial ; she must be their examiner, critic, interpreter, user, and judge. And no results of experiments can be made of any avail to medicine or be used with safety in her service until they have been filtered through the checks and counter-checks of clinical experience, and have responded to the tests and counter-tests of clinical trial. Had these principles exerted their just influence in the recent debates concerning questions of this kind, we should not have had a seton in the neck of a man taken as the parallel of a seton in the neck of a guinea-pig ; we should not have had the artificial tuberculosis of the rodent pronounced to be identical with the natural tuberculosis of a child ; we should not have had grey tubercles and caseous pneumonias pronounced, on the grounds of mere likeness of structure, to be of one and the same nature, and we should have been spared the sight of science, drunken with success and drivelling with prophecies, soliciting the public on the common highway."—*From* "*Abstract of an Address on Clinical Investigation*," "*British Medical Journal*," Feb. 3rd. 1883, pp. 191-192.

[Notwithstanding the above utterance, Sir A. Clark died a pro-vivisector.]

DEMONSTRATIONS TO STUDENTS. Purser.

JOHN MALLET PURSER, M.D., D.Sc., Professor of Institutes of Medicine, School of Physic, Trinity College, Dublin ; a witness before the Royal Commission of 1875. (V.)

(Q. 4,799A) : " Then do you contend for the powers of lecturers generally to perform painful operations for demonstration to students ?—Yes, I do." (Q. 4,827) : " In giving lectures in a private school, did you use demonstrations on living animals? —I did occasionally."—*Evid Roy. Com.* (London, 1876).

DEMONSTRATION—Repetition of painful Experiments for, unnecessary. Sharpey.

WILLIAM SHARPEY (the late), M.D., LL.D., F.R.S., formerly Professor of Physiology in King's College (born 1802 ; died 1880). (V.)

" I do not fully understand whether you justify painful experiments for the purpose of demonstration or not. Let me read this to you ; it is one of Dr. Michael Foster's chapters to illustrate this proposition, that ' the posterior roots are the channels of the centripetal (sensory), the anterior of centrifugal (motor) impulses,' to which you referred I think. ' Recurrent sensibility. This is never witnessed in the frog. It can only be shown in the higher animals, the cat or dog being best adapted for the purpose. The method adopted is very similar to the above. the arches of one or two vertebræ being carefully

H

sawn through or cut through with the bone forceps, and the
exposed roots being very carefully freed from the connective
tissue surrounding them. If the animal be strong and have
thoroughly recovered from the chloroform, and from the operation, irritation of the peripheral stump of the anterior root causes
not only contractions in the muscles supplied by the nerve,
but also movements in other parts of the body indicative of
pain or of sensations. On dividing the mixed trunk at some
little distance from the junction of the roots, the contractions
of the muscles supplied by the nerve cease, but the general
signs of pain or of sensation still remain.' I suppose that is a
well-established experiment, is it not; it is not one that is now
necessary?—Certainly I do not think it is necessary for exhibition at any rate."—*Evid Roy. Com.* (London, 1876), Q. 536.

DEMORALIZING EFFECTS of Demonstra-   Lister.
tions to Students.

SIR JOSEPH LISTER, M.B., F.R.C.S., Emeritus Professor of
Clinical Surgery, King's College, London. (V.)

"Attaches very great importance to demonstration as a
means of instruction (4,339-43). Considers that in class
demonstrations anæsthetics should be used, not so much
because it saves the animals pain, but because it prevents the
demoralizing effects of seeing unnecessary pain inflicted.
(4,328)."—*Digest of Evidence before Royal Commission* (London, 1876).

—— The same.   Haughton.

REV. SAMUEL HAUGHTON, D.D., F.R.S., Proctor, formerly
Medical Registrar, School of Physic, Trinity College, Dublin.
(A.V.)

"I would shrink with horror from accustoming classes of
young men to the sight of animals under vivisection. I believe
that many of them would become cruel and hardened, and
would go away and repeat these experiments recklessly
without foresight or forethought. Science would gain nothing,
and the world would have let loose upon it a set of young
devils.*—*Evid. Roy. Com.* (London, 1876), Q. 1.888.

---

* "By seeing these frequent experiments of one kind or another on living
animals, we tend to become brutalized and degraded, callous, and indifferent
to death or pain in others, and unfitted for our present work in the infirmary and
for future private practice."—*An Edinburgh Medical Student in " Scottish
Leader,"* Jan. 27th, 1890.

DEMORALIZING EFFECTS of Demonstrations to Students.   Acland.

HENRY WENTWORTH ACLAND, M.D., F.R.S. (afterwards Baronet), late Regius Professor of Medicine in the University of Oxford. (P.V.)

" So many persons have got to deal with these wonderful and beautiful organisms, just as they deal with physical bodies that have no feelings and no consciousness."—*Evid. Roy. Com.* (London. 1876), Q. 944.

—— The same.   Rolleston.

GEORGE ROLLESTON (the late). M.D. Oxon., 1857, F.R.C.P., F.R.S., Linacre Prof. of Anatomy at Oxford (born 1829 ; died 1890). (V.)

" Vivisection is specially likely to tempt a man into certain carelessness—the passive impressions produced by the sight of suffering growing, as is the law of our nature, weaker ; while the habit of, and the pleasure in, experimenting grows stronger by repetition."—*Evid. Roy. Com.* (London, 1876), Q. 1287.

—— The same.   Arnold.

F. S. ARNOLD, M.B., B.A. (Oxon), M.R.C.S., Manchester. (A.V.)

" The practice of vivisection seems to me absolutely incompatible with any true or high conception of the ἦθος of the medical profession. Our *rôle* is to save from suffering and death, not to inflict them. We have, of course, often to inflict suffering, but it is done with a view to save the individual from death or a greater suffering. We deal with patients, not with victims. The vivisector, on the other hand, inflicts suffering, not for the benefit of the sentient being on whom it is inflicted, but for the prospective benefit of another. *Qua* vivisector, he deals with victims. not with patients. I cannot see how it can be denied that the habitual dealing with victims, must have, at any rate, in many cases, a disastrous effect on the *morale* of the physician. How can we expect any but the most exceptional of men. to pass daily from the vivisectional laboratory to the hospital ward, and carry with them to the latter place none of the ideas and conceptions as to the rights of the individual which prevail in and govern the proceedings of the former ? I do not, of course, mean to charge all vivisectors with a neglect of the individual interests of their patients, but that the danger I have alluded to is real, is shown by the cancer-grafting experiments in Germany and France which horrified the world about a year ago."—*From a Paper read at the Church Congress, Folkestone,* 1892.

DIABETES AND VIVISECTION.   Berdoe.

EDWARD BERDOE, M R C.S., L.R.C.P.Ed., London.   (A.V.)

" Much light was thrown upon the cause of diabetes by Claude Bernard's discovery that injury to the floor of the lower part of the fourth ventricle of the brain caused sugar to appear in the urine.   Schiff discovered that section of the vaso-motor channels in a certain part of the spinal cord also caused this phenomenon.   Then Pavy and Eckhard pursued the inquiry on the same lines till the pathology and physiology of the matter became established.   Cyon also and others pursued a similar investigation with experiments on animals. Notwithstanding these important discoveries, interesting from a scientific aspect, *diabetes cannot be cured by them.*"— *Statement written by Dr. Berdoe,* Feb. 7th, 1894.

DIGITALIS—*See* FOXGLOVE LEAVES.

DIPHTHERIA, THE SERUM TREAT-   Hansemann.
MENT OF.

DR. HANSEMANN, Assistant to Professor Virchow, Berlin.   (V.).

" 1.   Löffler's bacillus not only appears in diphtheria cases, but also occurs in many healthy persons, and also in several kinds of slight disorders, such as catarrh of the *conjunctiva tunica.*   It is not therefore safe to consider it as the cause of diphtheria.

" 2.   The supposed effect of the serum in rendering human beings immune from diphtheria is not established.   Numerous cases of diphtheria have occurred notwithstanding the injection of the pretended immunizing serum.

" 3.   It is not a specific or a certain cure.   Even when injected on the first day of the attack, and in apparently slight cases, some children have died after the injections.   The statistics of the serum treatment are less favourable than those of some other modes of treatment.

" 4.   The serum remedy is not harmless, but produces dangerous skin diseases and sometimes fatal kidney inflammation." —*Substance of conclusions contained in a Paper read before the Medical Society of Berlin,* Nov. 29th, 1894.

DIPHTHERIA, THE SERUM TREAT-MENT OF.

Drasche.

PROFESSOR DRASCHE, Vienna. (P.V.)

" Professor Drasche's criticism was unfavourable to the new method, the effects of which he had had an opportunity of observing on some 30 cases in one of the Vienna hospitals. He found that the injections of the Behring anti-toxin serum affected the kidneys, and this observation was corroborated by those of other doctors. .... With regard to the statistics which were supposed to prove its success, Professor Drasche said that in diphtheria the bare figures were no evidence. He pointed out that, according to MM. Gottstein and Kassowitz, notwithstanding the use of the serum, the total mortality from diphtheria in Berlin and Vienna had not decreased. Clinical observation was the sole means by which a true judgment could be formed. In the 30 cases, the progress of which he had followed, he had not met a single instance in which he could feel convinced that the treatment had produced a direct effect. There were many symptoms which warned medical men against its use."—*Speech before the Vienna Medical Society*, " *Times*," London, Feb. 5th. 1895.

—— The same.

Kassowitz.

PROFESSOR KASSOWITZ, Vienna. (P.V.)

" Professor Kassowitz criticised in great detail the experimental observations upon which Behring had founded his method, and described them as insufficient in number and uncertain in teaching. He also expressed the opinion that the immunizing power of the serum could not be depended upon, and was, in fact, probably *nil*. He further laid stress on the fact that, as he believed, the serum had an injurious effect upon the heart, and that many cases had succumbed to heart failure, and pointed out that paralysis of the ocular muscles and of the extremities appeared to occur with greater frequency. He had used the serum in eight cases without observing any change in the temperature or pulse, or any definite improvement in the local conditions. He deprecated conclusions drawn from hospital statistics, since the mortality at different hospitals and in the same hospital at different times varied very much."—*Speech at Royal Medical Society, Vienna*, Jan. 18th, *reported in* " *British Medical Journal*," Feb. 16th, 1895.

DIPHTHERIA. STATISTICS OF THE SERUM TREATMENT.

"Medical Journal."

"THE BRITISH MEDICAL JOURNAL," Organ of the British Medical Association, London. (V.)

	B. M. J., Jan. 19th.		B. M. J., Feb. 2nd.		Treated Abroad.		Total.		
	Treated.	Died.	Treated.	Died.	Treated.	Died.	Treated.	Died.	Per-centage.
Under 1 year	12	6	4	2	2	1	18	9	50·00
1 to 2 years	34	11	9	3	18	6	61	20	32·78
2 ,, 3 ,, ...	27	8	6	1	14	3	47	12	25·53
3 ,, 4 ,, ...	23	3	12	1	8	—	43	4	9·30
4 ,, 5 ,, ...	26	8	10	3	13	2	49	13	26·53
5 ,, 10 ,, ...	37	2	23	9	21	3	81	14	17·28
10 ,, 15 ,, ...	13	—	15	2	7	—	35	2	5·71
Above 15 years	—	—	16	1	—	—	—	—	—
							334	74	22·10

—*British Medical Journal*, Feb. 16th, 1895, p. 386.

—— The same.   Moltchanoff.

V. A. MOLTCHANOFF, Schluessalburg. (P.V.)

This author "lays stress on the fact that the death-rate of epidemic diphtheria may oscillate without any relation whatever to the treatment employed, and that a low mortality was not unknown in the pre-serum days."—"*British Medical Journal*" (*quoting* "*Vratch*," Nov. 1st, 1895), Feb. 23rd, 1895, *Epitome*, p. 32.

—— The same. REMEDIES OTHER THAN SERUM.

"Journal de Médecine de Paris."

"JOURNAL DE MÉDECINE DE PARIS," edited by Dr. Lutaud, Paris. (R.)

"M. Lescure, physician to the Oran Hospital, with 40 per cent. solution of chromic acid, 54 cases, no death.

"M. Cutrin, with permanganate of potass, 2 per cent., 28 cases, in 8 of whom the bacillus of Löffler was identified, 7 deaths.

"M. Goubeau, sublimate of mercury and glycerine, 1 in 20, 21 cases, no death.

"M. Moizard, sublimate of mercury and glycerine, 173 cases, no death.

" M. Flatrault, raw petroleum, 15 cases, no death.
" M. Löffler, 96 cases, no death.
" De Crésantignes, Gaucher's method, 40 cases, 1 death.
" Total : 427 cases, 37 deaths, or a mortality of 8·66
per cent."—*Journal de Médecine de Paris*, Nov. 24th, 1894,
p. 567.

DIPHTHERIA. IMMUNISATION AGAINST.   Lebreton and Magdelaine.

MM. LEBRETON AND MAGDELAINE, Physicians, Hospital for
Sick Children, Paris. (P.V.)

" The authors conclude that the serum treatment is the one
to be preferred (*traitement de choix*) for diphtheria, but they
point out that the injections are not entirely harmless ; they
may cause rise of temperature and renal complications, and
in some cases a general condition that may, at least
transiently, give rise to some anxiety. They do not think,
therefore, as they were inclined to do at first, that prophylactic
injections should be given in the case of children who have
been exposed to infection."—"*British Medical Journal*," Feb.
23rd, 1895, p. 442 (*Report of paper read before Société Medicale
des Hopitaux*, Feb. 1st, 1895).

—— The same. IMMUNISATION : DEATH.   "Journal de Médecine de Paris."

"JOURNAL DE MÉDECINE DE PARIS," edited by Dr.
Lutaud, Paris. (R.)

" On the 15th January, Dr. Alfoldi was called to a female
child of eighteen months, suffering from diphtheria. He
injected 1,000 units of Behring's anti-toxin; on the fourth
day the false membranes had disappeared, and the child was
on the way to recovery. In the same bed with the child slept
a sister, aged three, and on January 18th the latter was
injected with the serum of Behring with the object of
immunising her against attack. The following day this second
child was prostrate, morose, and had no appetite. On the
morning of the 18th fever had set in, her temperature being
104·2. The child (a very intelligent one) complained of severe
pains in the loins, especially on the left side. On the 19th
the temperature was 104. During the night the body became
covered with a rash, and on the morning of the 20th death
supervened. Here was a case that must be considered, without
doubt, one of acute nephritis. The child was perfectly well

prior to the injection for the purpose of immunising it. and undoubtedly fell a victim to poisoning *(intoxication)* by the serum."—*Quoted from Prof. J. Kovach's Journal, "Gyogyaszot" (Buda Pesth) in the "Journal de Médecine de Paris,"* Feb. 24th, 1895, p. 111. *(See above.)*

DIPHTHERIA. VALUE OF SERUM AS   Woodhead. A REMEDY.

GERMAN SIMS WOODHEAD, M.D.Edin., Director of the Research Laboratory, Colleges of Phys. and Surgs., London. (V.)

" It should not be accepted that this agent can reduce the cure of diphtheria to a mere process of injection. Everything must be done to improve the conditions under which the patients are treated, to maintain their strength. to give them fresh air, cleanly surroundings, and good general hygienic conditions. It will be found withal that a certain number of deaths from rapid poisoning will take place, while a number of others will succumb in the later stages of the disease. This serum can no more act as a specific in every case than can quinine cure every case of malaria. . . The antitoxic serum treatment is only one of our lines of defence against this disease."—*Extract from a Lecture delivered at the Royal Institution,* Feb. 8th, 1895.

—— The same.   "Saturday Review."

" THE SATURDAY REVIEW," London Weekly Newspaper. (N.)

"To judge from the assiduity with which the leading London papers have puffed the alleged anti-toxin cure for diphtheria, it would seem that the medical profession has at length discovered how sweet are the uses of—advertisement. It is a pity, however, that the English press should continue to be made the catspaw of a gang of foreign medical adventurers, and this consideration has induced us to set before them and the public at large a few facts concerning the statistics of diphtheria and the pretensions of these gentlemen." —*"The Saturday Review,"* Feb. 2nd, 1895.

DISEASE—Vivisection has done very little   Crisp. good in the treatment of.

EDWARD CRISP, M.D., a witness before the Royal Commission, 1875. (A.V.)

"I am rather penitent in this matter. I have been a

vivisector for some time, and as I advanced in age, and I hope
in wisdom, I saw fit to alter my opinion. . . . I have also
come to the conclusion that, in a practical point of view, very
little good has resulted from vivisection as regards the treatment of disease. . . . The cerebellum has been sliced in
all directions and in various ways, and various conclusions, as
is well known, have been drawn—very opposite conclusions
indeed. . . . I believe the advocates of vivisection have
very much exaggerated the good resulting from it."—*Evid.
Roy. Com.* (London. 1876), Q. 6,157 and 6,159.

DOMINION, MAN'S, A MORAL TRUST.—*See* MORAL TRUST.

DONERAILE, LORD, CASE OF.—*See* HYDROPHOBIA, M. Pasteur and Lord Doneraile's Case.

DOUBTFUL RESULTS OF VIVISECTION.   Rutherford.

RUTHERFORD, WILLIAM, M.D.Edin.; M.R.C.S.Eng.; Professor of Institutes of Medicine, Edinburgh University. (V.)

"In your judgment and your own experience, are operations
of that description upon a dog to be taken as being evidence
of what the effect would be on the human being?—Certainly
not, but merely as suggesting what the action would be; that
is all. The experiment must also be tried upon man before
a conclusion can be drawn."—*Evid. Roy. Com.* (London, 1876),
Q. 2,966.

DROWNING, Futile Experiments as to.   Macaulay.

JAMES MACAULAY, M.A., M.D., F.R.C.S.Ed., London. (A.V.)

"I do not know any more striking example of the futile
results of experimental inquiry than that which was instituted
some years ago on suspended animation. The Royal Humane
Society had received from Dr. Silvester, and other medical
men, various suggestions as to the best mode of treating
persons apparently drowned. The Committee referred the
proposals to the Royal Medical and Chirurgical Society, with
a request for advice. A committee of investigation was
appointed by the Royal Medical and Chirurgical Society,
consisting of the following members:—C. J. B. Williams,
M.D., F.R.S.; C. E. Brown-Séquard, M.B., F.R.S.; George
Harley, M.D., W. S. Kirkes, M.D.; H. Hyde Salter, M.D.,
F.R.S.; J. Burdon-Sanderson, M.D.; W. S. Savory, F.R.S.;
and E. H. Sieveking, M.D.

❋   ❋   ❋

" In pursuing the inquiry, a large number of experiments were made upon living animals. In the first place, the phenomena of apnœa 'suffocation], in its least complicated form, were investigated—viz., when produced by simply depriving the animal of air. Tracheotomy was performed upon animals fastened down to a table on their backs, and glass tubes inserted, and secured firmly by ligature. Through a tube thus inserted the animal could breathe freely, but the air could be at once and effectively cut off by inserting a tightly-fitting cork into the upper end of the tube. In this way a measure could be obtained of the time when respiration would cease. In order to observe in the same animals the duration of the action of the heart, long pins were inserted through the thoracic walls into some part of the ventricles. The movements of the pin indicated the motion of the heart after the cardiac sounds had ceased to be audible. The conclusions from many experiments was that, in simple apnœa, the action of the heart continued a considerable time after the respiratory movements had ceased,—a fact well known, and needing no cruel experiments to establish it."— *Vivisection : A Prize Essay* (London, 1881), pp. 57-8.

DROWNING.   Macaulay.
JAMES MACAULAY, M.A., M.D., F.R.C.S.Ed., London.   (A.V.)

"On proceeding to experiments on drowning, it was found that the time of possible recovery of dogs, after immersion, was only 1 minute 30 seconds, on an average, instead of 4 minutes, from simple deprivation of air. ' To what is this striking difference due ? ' the investigators ask. Experiments were made in order to eliminate from the inquiry the element of struggling, also the element of cold, and, lastly, the access of water to the lungs. On this latter point it was found that a dog with the windpipe plugged recovered from a longer sub-mersion than a dog without the windpipe plugged.

    *   *   *   *   *

" In presenting their report to the Royal Humane Society, the Royal Medical and Chirurgical Society were able to recommend no practical suggestions as the result of their inquiry. —*Vivisection : A Prize Essay* (London, 1881), p. 59.

DRUGS, Different effects of, on Animals   Berdoe.
and Man.
EDWARD BERDOE, M.R.C.S., L.R.C.P.Ed., London.   (A.V.)

" It has long been a familiar fact to those who protest

against the practices of vivisection, that there are several drugs which are deadly poisons to man which are eaten with impunity by goats, rabbits, and other mammals; for instance, goats eat hemlock, and take no harm; rabbits devour belladonna with impunity; pigeons are not affected by doses of opium strong enough to kill a man."—*The Futility of Experiments with Drugs on Animals*, by Edward Berdoe (London, 1889), pp. 4, 5.

DRUGS. Bochefontaine.

LOUIS THEODORE BOCHEFONTAINE, late Prof. Experimental Pathology, Medical Faculty, Paris. (V.)

" All the experiments which we describe on this subject have been made on dogs and on a cat. Some few which are not mentioned were made on rabbits and a few on guinea-pigs. The results obtained amount to little or nothing. We must say once for all that our experiments with strychnine and quinine have also given no exact result."—*Collection de Thèses pour le Doctorat* (Paris, 1873), p. 25.

" . . . Even in the same species of animals, though the experimenters act under identical conditions, the results obtained are not always the same."—*Ibid.*, p. 33.

—— The same. Bowie.

JOHN BOWIE, L.R.C.P., L.R.C.S., Edinburgh. (A.V.)

" That the physiologists have not been contemplating the laws of being, or rendering more effective our dealing with disease, is substantiated by the indisputable fact that, during the past two thousand years—the period claimed by the vivisectors as that in which experiments have been performed on man and the lower creation—there has not been discovered by them the action of one drug for the cure of a single disease. Our adversaries proclaim to the world a delusion, and many have accepted as matter of fact that which is positively untrue."—*Reply to Dr. Rutherford*, Dec. 24, 1880 (*Review* Office, 20, St. Giles' Street, Edinburgh), p. 24.

—— The same. Bowie.

JOHN BOWIE, L.R.C.P., L.R.C.S., Edinburgh. (A.V.)

" Through a long series of years, philosophic and clear-sighted physicians in various regions of the globe have been studiously engaged in examining into the actions and uses of such remedies as aconite, belladonna, antimony, strychnine, mercury, digitalis, arsenic, quinine, opium, henbane, and a long list of drugs from the mineral and vegetable kingdoms, too numerous to mention—inflicting no pain on any animal, but with the best and happiest results. There is, therefore, no need for a single painful experiment being executed to discover the remedial properties, actions, and uses of medicines. The mode in which vivisectionists get up their experiments and discoveries is a perfect fraud upon science."—*Reply to Dr. Rutherford*, Dec. 24, 1880 (*Review* Office, 20, St. Giles' Street, Edinburgh), p. 18.

DRUGS.   Watson.

SIR THOMAS WATSON, BART., M.D. (the late), Past President Royal College of Physicians (born 1792 ; died 1866). (V.)

" LORD WINMARLEIGH : Does it follow that because any drug would be poisonous to a dog it would necessarily be poisonous to a man ?—No, not at all. On that account I think it was that you said that you had no great faith in experiments made of the effects of drugs upon animals ?—No, I should not have any faith in such experiments."—*Evid. Roy. Com.* (London, 1876), Q. 57-8.

—— The same. Discovery of Chloral.   Clarke.

JOHN H. CLARKE, M.D., Physician to the Homœopathic Hospital, London. (A.V.)

" ' Philanthropos ' next gives us a list of medicines, the virtues of which were all discovered, according to our author, by vivisections. Among these is chloral. We notice this because so much was made of it by Virchow in his celebrated address in 1881, and because it affords a good example of the danger of taking laboratory evidence as to the powers and actions of drugs. We have not yet had the details given us as to how the virtues of this drug became known, but this we do know, that on its first appearance it was lauded as being equal to opium as a hypnotic, and without any of its after effects or any of its risks. We were assured that there was no danger of chloral gaining power over those who took it so as to render them slaves of a habit. Accordingly it became the fashion ; and soon its hundreds of victims proved how false the deductions from the teaching of the laboratory had been. How, indeed, could it be learned there whether or not chloral had power over the moral being of man ? It was impossible. Chloral madness became a not unfrequent disease ; and the victims whom it kept in slavery without reducing to madness were, and are, still more numerous."—*Physiological Cruelty ; a reply to " Philanthropos "* (London, 1883), p. 43.

DRUGS. Pritchard.

WILLIAM PRITCHARD, M.R.C.V.S. (the late), Professor of Anatomy, Royal Veterinary College. (A.V.)

" I do not think that the use of drugs on animals can be taken as a guide as to the doses or the action of the same drugs on human subjects; and, therefore, I do not think they are instructive, or only to a slight extent. . . . They cannot be depended upon."—*Evid. Roy. Com.* (London, 1876), pp.908-9.

—— Claimed by Vivisectors as given to Medicine by Vivisection. Harris.

STANFORD HARRIS, M.R.C.S., London. (A.V.)

List by Dr. Yeo in the Arris and Gale Lectures at the Royal College of Surgeons : —
Chloral Hydrate.
The antagonism between Atropia and Calabar Bean.
Amyl Nitrite.
Nux Vomica and the antagonism between its active principle (strychnine) and tobacco.
The effect of carbolic acid in checking the formation of sugar in diabetes.
Answer by Mr. Stanford Harris, being part of a lecture given at the High School, Manchester, to the Association of School Teachers:—
"Chloral Hydrate was introduced into practice by Dr. Liebrich. It was the fact that alkalies caused this chemical to be converted into chloroform that suggested to him the idea of its possible use in medicine " (*Wood's Therapeutics*, p. 290). 'This discovery reminds us of the similar one of the discovery of the use of chloroform by Sir James Simpson, who tried the effect upon himself" (*English Blue Book on Vivisection*, 2,595). " The discovery was established and then vivisection followed. Respecting the value of experiments on the lower animals with chloral, I may refer to Dr. Yeo himself, Langley, and others in the *British Medical Journal* and *Lancet* to the effect that 60 grains of croton chloral will send a dog to sleep for two hours only, while for man the dose is one-sixth of that amount. In fact, Dr. Ringer's experiments on animals in the case of another drug, nitrite of sodium, lead him to state in his book to practitioners, the dose of nitrite of sodium to be 20 grains, a dose which he afterwards explained in a letter to the *Lancet* (November 17, 1883) was a dangerous one, the right dose being 3 grains. Query, how many practitioners had in the meantime

administered the dose recommended, and how many human patients had been put into danger in consequence ?

"The antagonism between Atropia and Calabar Bean is again a case of vivisection *following* a discovery. A German doctor (Dr. Kleinwächter) in 1864 successfully treated a case of poisoning by atropia with calabar bean ; and in 1867, a Frenchman (Dr. Bonneville), commenced his experiments on animals, followed by a Scotchman (Dr. Fraser), who experimented on 331 rabbits to prove what had been proved three years before in actual practice " (*Wood's Therapeutics*, p. 276).

"Amyl Nitrite was introduced by Dr. B. W. Richardson in 1865. The experiments of Dr. Gamgee some years later are claimed as the foundation of its use in medicine. It relieves, but does not cure, certain cases of angina pectoris, or spasm of the heart. Now none can handle a bottle of nitrite of amyl for two minutes without having its effects demonstrated upon his face. It dilates the blood-vessels. The fact could not fail to be known to each physician to whose notice Dr. Richardson had introduced it previous to Dr. Gamgee's experiments. Now when Dr. Lauder Brunton was looking out for a dilator of the blood-vessels to relieve angina pectoris, here was one to his hand. In the words of Dr. McCormick, Deputy-Inspector of Hospitals and Fleets in England, 'the fact that amyl nitrite often relieves angina pectoris could have been very readily arrived at by letting a patient inhale its vapours. Animal torture was unnecessary.'

"Similarly, the antidotal powers of tobacco in poisoning by strychnine are falsely given as a discovery due to vivisection. A host of vivisections, as in all similar cases, followed the fact that tobacco had cured a case of strychnine poisoning. I remember that when a student, during the course of lectures given by Dr. Somers to us in 1872, our lecturer having no anti-vivisectionists in his mind, and not being aware how soon such sentimentalists, as they are called, would come into existence, graphically describing the case, where tobacco had been first tried in strychnine poisoning. He told us that a case occurring in the practice of an American doctor, he was struck by the idea that as his suffering patient was being convulsed through overaction of the spinal cord, he might try tobacco, which he knew from experience caused paralysis of the cord in large doses. It was tried, and succeeded. However, I may mention that the later books omit tobacco as an advisable antidote, chloroform being the best antidotal action " (*Dr. Ringer's Therapeutics*). "In fact, we are warned that the treatment of tobacco is a somewhat dangerous one,

because while paralysing the cord it may also stop the heart "
(*Wood's Therapeutics*, p. 264).

" Respecting the employment of Carbolic Acid as an internal
remedy, the fact that small doses can be so taken is not new.
Having been tried for zymotic and other diseases, to quote
Wood, ' the study of its physiological action has failed to show
the possession of any property which should render the
medicine valuable in constitutional diseases, and clinical
experience has borne this out : so that it is employed directly
in medicine only for its local effects. I quote this to show
that carbolic acid has been extensively tried on the human
being, and, therefore, if for diabetes or any other complaint, it was thought desirable to try carbolic, the way
was open. Let me illustrate what I mean by a supposed
case. If it were suggested that quinine would be likely to
cure a particular skin disease, it would be merely necessary
to try it upon the sufferer, because the fact that quinine
is a chemical safe to administer to the human subject is
well known. But if, instead of this, animals had quinine
injected into their brains, livers, and other organs, by some
zealous vivisector, then we should be told that vivisection had
enabled quinine to be tried in this particular case."

DRUGS, Pain caused by Experiments with.   Wood.

GEO. B. WOOD, M.D., LL.D. (the late), an American Medical
Man. (V.)

" As I have seen the rabbit after the injection of one-sixth
or one-quarter grain of Mason's pure aconitia, the animal
commences to jump vertically in a very peculiar manner, and
often to squeal piteously. The jumping soon grows less
and less powerful, and finally is replaced by severe convulsions."—*Wood's Therapeutics*, p. 149.

DUTY TO MAN AND DUTY TO BEAST.—*See* MORAL
ASPECTS, COBBE, MACKARNESS.

ECRASEUR, The.   Tait.

LAWSON TAIT, F.R.C.S., late Professor of Gynæcology, Queen's
College, Birmingham. (A.V.)

" Mr. Gamgee quotes the introduction of the ecraseur as an
instance of the influence of vivisection on the progress of
human surgery. No more unfortunate instance could be
quoted. The principle of the instrument is that it crushes and

tears the tissues instead of cutting them as by the knife. The surgical aphorism that 'torn arteries don't bleed' was in existence long before M. Chassaignac was born, and if he had based his employment on that alone he could have done all that his instrument has effected. But unfortunately he performed experiments upon animals, and immediately he was led astray. I once saw the leg of a favourite dog amputated at the hip joint on account of disease, and when the limb was removed not a single vessel bled, and the main artery was tied only as a matter of precaution. In the human subject I have seen twelve or fifteen arteries tied in the same operation, for with us the smallest arteries bleed and require to be secured. Our arteries act in ways altogether different from those seen in the lower animals. Their pathology and physiology are absolutely different, as may be seen in the frequency of apoplexy and aneurism with us, and the almost complete immunity from them of all the lower animals, even in extreme old age. Hunter tried his best to induce aneurism to the lower animals, and failed. Injuries to arteries in the lower animals are repaired with the utmost certainty and readiness, but in man it is altogether different. It may be easily imagined, therefore, that M. Chassaignac's application of the ecraseur to the lower animals was found wholly misleading when man was the subject, and now in human surgery its utility is extremely limited; that is, it is entirely confined to operations where only very small arteries are divided. Speaking for my own practice, I may say that it might be dispensed with and never missed."—*Uselessness of Vivisection*, by Lawson Tait (Birmingham, 1882). pp. 33-4.

ELATERIUM.   Berdoe.

EDWARD BERDOE, M.R.C.S., F.R.C.P.Ed., London.   (A.V.)

"This drug, even in very small doses, causes in man violent purging, with severe griping, and more or less vomiting; but, however it may be given to dogs and rabbits, does not vomit or purge them, but destroys them with tetanoid phenomena. (*Stillé and Maisch*, p. 521.)"—*The Futility of Experiments with Drugs on Animals*, by Edward Berdoe (London, 1889), p. 19.

EPILEPSY Produced on Animals,   Althaus.
unlike the Human Malady.

JULIUS ALTHAUS, M.D., Consulting Physician to the Epileptic Hospital, London.   (V.)

"A form of epilepsy may be caused in guinea-pigs which, in

some respects, resembles human epilepsy and has even been transmitted to the offspring of the animals ; yet it has the tendency to disappear spontaneously, without the aid of digitalis or bromide of potassium, and is, after all, by no means the actual disease with which we are familiar in our patients."— *British Medical Journal* (June 4th, 1881), p. 873.

EPILEPSY.—*See* NERVES, THE REFLEX ACTION OF THE.

ERROR, Vivisection, A Source of.—*See* MISLEADING, etc.

ETHER.   " Provincial Medical Journal."

"THE PROVINCIAL MEDICAL JOURNAL, " Edited by Dr. Dolan, Published at Leicester. (N.)

"William Thomas Green Morton, M.D., medical student, dentist and physician, and the recent recipient of Massachusetts' honour, was born in Charlton, Mass., August 9th, 1819, and died, aged forty eight, in New York City, July 5th, 1868. . . . "On September 30th, 1846, at his office in Boston, he administered sulphuric ether to Eben Frost and extracted a tooth without pain to the patient.

" Securing permission from Dr. John C. Warren, Senior Surgeon of the Massachusetts General Hospital, on October 16th, 1846, he administered ether to a patient at the hospital, and Dr. Warren performed a severe surgical operation, the patient remaining unconscious during the operation. . . .

" From this crucial demonstration in October, 1846, dates the immediate and universal adoption of the practice of anæsthesia throughout the civilized world. The event marked the advent of a new epoch in the world's history, namely, the epoch of practical painless surgery.

" Over Dr. Morton's grave in Mount Auburn Cemetery, near Boston, a monument has been erected by citizens of Boston, including names the most respected and most honoured among them, bearing the following inscription, written by the late Dr. Jacob Bigelow, of Boston : 'William T. G. Morton, inventor and revealer of anæsthetic inhalation, by whom pain in surgery was averted and annulled. Before whom, in all time, surgery was agony. Since whom science has control of pain.' "—*Extracts from " Provincial Medical Journal,"* April, 1895, p. 201.

—— **The same.**   **Gimson.**

W. GIMSON GIMSON, M.D., M.R.C.S., Witham, Essex.   (A.V.)

" Ether came next into use about 1846, travelling to us from

I

America. ' It was employed in every variety of surgical operation, from Cæsarean section, in which it was used by Mr. Skey, at St. Bartholomew's Hospital, on the 25th of January, 1847, down to tooth-drawing. It was used to tranquilise the insane, to detect feigned disease, and to diminish the sufferings incidental to parturition.' "—*Vivisections and Painful Experiments on Living Animals* (London, 1879), pp. 128.

ETHER. CHLORIC.   Gimson.

W. GIMSON GIMSON, M.D., M.R.C.S., Witham, Essex.   (A.V.)

" In the summer of 1847, Michael Cudmore Furnell, then a student of St. Bartholomew's Hospital, was residing in the house of Bell & Co., of Oxford Street, to perfect himself in practical pharmacy. Excited by the recent discovery of ether, he made many experiments on the different varieties of inhalers. One day, whilst looking for *sulphuric* ether, he found a dusty bottle labelled ' *Chloric Ether*.' He boldly experimented on *himself*, and inhaled some of this liquid, which produced a certain amount of insensibility without the suffocating irritation and choking caused by ether. He communicated his observation to Mr. Holmes Coote, who used the compound during several operations performed by Lawrence, in the summer of 1847. But whilst Furnell, Lawrence, and Holmes Coote did not get beyond the observation of the fact, and did not know that chloric ether was an alcholic solution of chloroform, Simpson not only discovered, but identified and investigated the properties of chloroform, published his discoveries and established its use. (*Druitt's Surgeon's Vade Mecum*)."—*Vivisections and Painful Experiments on Living Animals* (London, 1879), pp. 128–9.

—— **The same.**—*See also* ANÆSTHETICS.

EXPERIMENTER FATALLY INFECTED.—*See* TUBERCULOSIS, "GAULOIS."

EXPERIMENTS, NATURE'S   Murray.

WILLIAM MURRAY, M.D., F.R.C.P., Lond., M.R.C.S., Lauréat de l'Acad. Méd., Paris, Physician to out-patients, Westminster Hospital, London. (P.V.)

" In disease nature is for ever making fresh experiments before our eyes, and we are to watch how she varies the experiment, lest its many variations from the normal type of the disease mislead us into a false diagnosis. Each disease varies as much in expression as the human countenance. In my experience no two cases are exactly alike. What is described as a typical case exists only in the imagination of the writer of a text-book or a lecturer to his class."—"*The Lancet*," *Vol.* I., 1892, p. 1021.

EXPERIMENTS, ENGLISH. Brunton.

THOMAS LAUDER BRUNTON, M.D.Edin., F.R.C.P.Lond., Lecturer on Materia Medica and Therapeutics, St. Bartholomew's Hospital, London. (V.)

" Dr. Lauder Brunton, Professor at St. Bartholomew's Hospital, records in *The Practitioner*, for October, 1884, a series of experiments on Febrile Temperature, by himself and Dr. Cash. One cat, *e.g.* was subjected to such a temperature as sufficed to raise its *internal* heat to 115·8° Fahr. How great must have been the *external* heat necessary to do this through its heat-resisting fur, we can scarcely imagine. The animals were fixed so that they could not move ; the vagi nerves were cut and stimulated, and the digitalis was injected under their skin, their temperatures being carefully taken all the time they were dying, as we are told, from ' hyperpyrexia '—which,being interpreted, is over-heat,or in a word.baking."—See *Practitioner*, October, 1884.

—— The same.—*See also* ACT, THE, EXPERIMENTS UNDER.

EXPERIMENTS, The More the Better. Lankester.

EDWIN RAY LANKESTER, M.A., M.D., F.R.S. Professor of Anatomy (Linacre), Oxford. (V.)

" If you allow experiment at all, you must admit the more of it the better, since it is certain that for many years to come the problems of physiology demanding experimental solution will increase in something like geometrical ratio instead of decreasing."—*Letter in the* " *Spectator*," Jan. 10th, 1874.

—— The same, Tens of Thousands of.—*See* RESULTS—Macaulay.

FALLACIOUSNESS of the Results of Gimson. Vivisection.

W. GIMSON GIMSON, M.D., F.R.C.S., Witham, Essex. (A.V.)

·' We are more especially concerned with experiments which are *painful* in their performance. The qualification of itself, at once suggests two grounds for fallacy in the prosecution of any such inquiry, viz. the disturbance caused by the pain if sensation is allowed to exist ; and the derangement of the whole system if sensation is overcome by the use of anæsthetics."—*Vivisections and Painful Experiments on Living Animals : their Unjustifiability* (London, 1879), p. 59.

FEELINGS, The, of Vivisectors blunted.   Hoggan.

GEORGE HOGGAN, M.D. (the late), a witness before the Royal Commission of 1875 (born 1837 ; died 1891). (A.V.)

" Were the feelings of experimental physiologists not blunted they could not long continue the practice of vivisection. They are always ready to repudiate any implied want of tender feeling, but I must say that they seldom show much pity ; on the contrary, in practice they frequently show the reverse. Hundreds of times I have seen, when an animal writhed with pain, and thereby deranged the tissues, during a delicate dissection, instead of being soothed it would receive a slap and an angry order to be quiet and to behave itself. At other times, when an animal had endured great pain for hours without struggling or giving more than an occasional low whine, instead of letting the poor mangled wretch loose to crawl painfully about the place in reserve for another day's torture, it would receive pity so far that it would be said to have behaved well enough to merit death ; and, as a reward, would be killed at once by breaking up the medulla with a needle, or 'pithing,' as this operation is called. I have heard the Professor say, when one side of an animal had been so mangled and the tissues so obscured by clotted blood that it was difficult to find the part searched for, ' Why don't you begin on the other side ? ' or, ' Why don't you take another dog ? ' ' What is the use of being so economical ? ' "—*From an article by Dr. Hoggan, in " Fraser's Magazine,"* April, 1875.

FERRIER, Prosecution of Professor,   Cobbe.
why it failed.

FRANCES POWER COBBE, Authoress, Hengwrt, Dolgelly. (A.V.)

" Mr. Cartwright twitted Mr. Reid for not alluding to the prosecution of Professor Ferrier. He said that that prosecution ' lamentably broke down. The charge brought against Dr. Ferrier was that he operated without a licence and infringed the law by doing those things to which the hon. and learned Member referred, but the charge was not supported by one tittle of evidence.'

" The ' tittle of evidence ' on which the charge of the Victoria Street Society against Professor Ferrier was supported was simply the direct and repeated statements of the two leading medical papers in London—the *Lancet* and the *British Medical Journal*—viz. that Dr. Ferrier had exhibited in King's College, and in the presence of one hundred members of the Medical Congress, certain monkeys on which he had performed his well-known experiments. As the Home Office replied to the Society's inquiries that Professor Ferrier had no licence authorizing him to perform those experiments, the legal advisers of the Victoria Street Society naturally thought that they had a clear case of infraction of the law. But what was the ' break down ' of the case wherein Mr. Cartwright triumphed, and on whom did it throw discredit? Both the medical papers, as we have said, attributed the experiments in question to Professor Ferrier. They stated that 'the animals were monkeys on which Professor Ferrier had operated some months previously,' and which ' Professor Ferrier was willing to exhibit; ' that they were ' exhibited by Professor Ferrier.' These statements had remained for four months without any modification or correction. Yet when the prosecution took place the Editor of the *British Medical Journal* brought his reporter, Dr. Roy, into Court to swear point-blank that he had made a mistake in attributing the experiments to Professor Ferrier, who had nothing to do with the experiments ; and that from first to last they had been to his knowledge the work of somebody else, to wit, Professor Yeo. The reporter of the *Lancet* was not in Court ; but when the prosecution proposed an adjournment for his examination, Professor Ferrier's counsel stated, in the presence of the Editor of the *Lancet*, that he had communicated with that reporter, and that he was prepared to swear the same as Dr. Roy.

" Now, assuming, as we are bound to do, that this was not perjury on the part of the medical journal's staff and of Professor Michael Foster, who swore likewise that the experiments were performed by Professor Yeo, there are only two hypotheses open—

" Either, *first*, Dr. Roy, in his draft report of the experiments he had just witnessed, attributed them rightly to ' Professor Yeo,' and then the Editor, for some occult reason, substituted, throughout, the name of ' Ferrier ' for ' Yeo.'

" Or, *second*, Dr. Roy wrote ' Ferrier,' by mistake, all through a long report, when he meant ' Yeo ' ; and (wonderful to relate !) Professor Gamgee, in reporting for the *Lancet*, underwent precisely the same very remarkable hallucination.

" We should have imagined—our legal advisers imagined—
that the harmonious elaborate reports of experiments by the
two great organs of the medical profession, afforded something
more than a 'tittle of evidence' on the matter; but the upshot
certainly justified Mr. Cartwright's denial that there *was* a
'tittle of evidence' against Professor Ferrier. Only it may be
questioned whether the 'breakdown' of a case under such
circumstances, ought to be felt most 'lamentable' by the
prosecutors, who believed in the substantial veracity of the
medical organs; or by the defendants, who escaped by a
process more nearly resembling thimble-rigging than is
commonly witnessed in English courts of justice. 'Who
do you think, gentlemen, we have got under this cup?'
'Why, Professor Ferrier, to be sure! We saw him put there
by the *Lancet* and the *British Medical Journal*.' 'I think you
are mistaken, gentlemen,' says the *prestidigitateur*, as he raises
the cup; and lo! there in sooth, is Professor Yeo!"—
Comments on the Debate in the House of Commons, April 4th,
1883, by Frances Power Cobbe (London, 1883), pp. 2-4.

FERRIER PROSECUTION, The. The Sequel.   Ferrier.

DAVID FERRIER, M.D., F.R.S., Professor of Neuropathy, King's
College, London. (V.)

" The facts recorded in this paper are partly the results of
a research made conjointly by Drs. Ferrier and Yeo, aided by
a grant from the British Medical Association, and partly of a
research made by Dr. Ferrier alone, aided by a grant from the
Royal Society, and 'the *conjoint experiments* are distinguished
by an asterisk.' "—*Prefatory Note to* " *A Record of Experiments
on the Effect of Lesion of Different Regions of the Cerebral
Hemispheres,*" by David Ferrier, M.D., and Gerald F. Yeo,
M.D., read January 24th, 1884. (See second part of the *Philosophical Transactions of the Royal Society for* 1884).

FLIES AND THE DIFFUSION OF   " Medical
BACTERIA.   Journal."

"THE BRITISH MEDICAL JOURNAL," Organ of the British
Medical Association. (V.)

Dr. Simmonds's investigations on the transportation of
cholera bacilli by flies are of interest in that they give in
the form of a definite experimental observation what has
long been almost common knowledge. It is well known that
flies that have access to tuberculous sputum take the tubercle

bacilli into their intestines. If they are examined histologically some time after, these bacilli may be demonstrated with the utmost readiness by the ordinary methods. . . Dr. Simmonds placed a number of flies which had from time to time settled on the viscera, etc., of a cholera case on which he was performing a *post-mortem* examination in a flask large enough to allow of their free movement. As soon as they had been moving about long enough to ensure their having got rid of most extraneous particles (about three-quarters of an hour), they were placed in a tube containing a suitable nutrient gelatine, from which plate cultures were made. In a couple of days these plates were covered with colonies of the cholera bacillus, and the proof was complete.—" *British Medical Journal*," December 2nd, 1893. p. 1236.

FLIES AND THE DIFFUSION OF BACTERIA. Berdoe.

EDWARD BERDOE, M.R.C.S. Eng., L.R.C.P. Ed., London (A.V.)

"I was shown over the (Pasteur) laboratories, and there I saw in long glass tubes the cultures of multiform diseases. But glass will break in the best regulated rooms, and then it is thrown into a common zinc pail without a cover, and the cultures in jelly are taken at "discretion" by the "busy curious thirsty flies," who, not being vertebrate animals, visit the torture chambers of science fearless and free."—*From the* " *Echo*," *London*, September 19th, 1894.

—— The same. " The Times."

"THE TIMES," London Daily Newspaper. (P.V.)

"Mr. W. T. Burgess exhibited the result of rather an alarming experiment, from which it would seem that flies which have been exposed to infection may convey it to potatoes by simply walking over them."—" *Royal Society Conversazione*," "*Times*," May 2nd, 1889 p. 7, col. 2.

FLIES.—*See also* CHOLERA AND FLIES.

FLY AGARIC, or Fly Fungus (Fungus muscarius), Contradictions of Experiments with. Berdoe.

EDWARD BERDOE, M.R.C.S., L.R.C.P.Ed., London. (A.V.)

"This poisonous fungus yields the deadly alkaloid *Muscarine*. In commenting upon a case of poisoning by this fungus, related by Dr. Chevers, Stillé says (p. 664), 'in this narrative there is absolutely nothing to suggest, or to be explained by the results of the physiological experiments above described.' They never do explain anything which is of any importance.

"Ringer and Morshead found that muscarine *dilated* the pupil when applied locally.

" Schmiedeberg and Harnack discovered that it *contracted* the pupil both when applied locally and given internally.— (Brunton, *Materia Medica*, p. 187.)"—*The Futility of Experiments with Drugs on Animals*, by Edward Berdoe (London, 1889), p. 20.

FOXGLOVE LEAVES (*Digitalis*).   Berdoe.

EDWARD BERDOE, M.R.C.S., L.R.C.P.Ed., London. (A.V.)

" This drug is perhaps the most valuable one which we possess for the treatment of certain forms of heart disease. It has often been claimed by our opponents of the experimental school that its virtues were discovered in consequence of the great number of investigations which have been carried out with it upon the lower animals. But this is a typical case of the confusion so often made between a discovery and its demonstration. 'Long before' (we quote from Stillé's great work, p. 511) 'its mode of action had been experimentally investigated, it was established as the most efficient remedy for dropsy depending upon disease of the heart, or upon that form of renal disease which consists of congestion and tubal obstruction.' . . . Great confusion exists among experimenters as to its action upon the heart. Its action upon the kidneys has been studied by numerous observers with diverse results. With reference to its influence on the blood pressure, note the following quotations :—

" ' Boehm, experimenting with digitalis, found that under certain anatomical conditions it does not increase arterial pressure.'—(*Wood*, p. 138.)

" ' The rise in blood pressure is regarded by Schmiedeberg, Boehm, and others, as entirely due to increased action of the heart, and not to contraction of the vessels.' — (*Brunton*, p. 911.)

" ' Ackerman, under precisely similar circumstances, found the direct opposite.'—(*Wood*, p. 139.)

" ' With this view I cannot agree, and I still hold to the opinion which I expressed many years ago, that the rise in pressure is due in great measure to the contraction of the arterioles.'—(*Brunton, loc. cit.*)"—*The Futility of Experiments with Drugs on Animals*, by Edward Berdoe (London, 1889), pp. 20-21.

FRUITLESSNESS OF VIVISECTION.   Garretson.

JAMES GARRETSON, M.D., Philadelphia, U.S.A.   (A.V.)

" If anything specially new or good has been evolved from vivisection which could not equally well have been learned after another manner, I do not know it.

✢   ✢   ✢   ✳   ✢

" Human beings would lose *nothing*."—*Address at Phila-delphia*, 1885.

FUTILITY OF EXPERIMENTS.—*See* DROWNING.

GADARENE SWINE, THE.   Bell.

ERNEST BELL, London.   (A.V.)

" The story of the Gadarene swine, so often appealed to by vivisectors as evidence in favour of their practice, is clearly misunderstood by them. It is so like a vivisector to put himself without a moment's hesitation in the place of the Deity. But in the analogy—if analogy there is any at all—the vivisectors are in the position, not of Christ, but of the devils, whom He permitted to torment the swine at their own request, for the same inscrutable reason, possibly, that the vivisectors and other cruel people are allowed now to torment animals for their own ends.' "—E. B.

GALVANI AND THE FROGS.   Cobbe.

FRANCES POWER COBBE, Authoress, Hengwrt, Dolgelly.   (A.V.)

" Dr. Playfair spoke of the time when Galvani ' put a copper hook through the spine of *live* frogs and hung them on the iron rails of his balcony in Bologna.'

" ' The lover sees the beloved object everywhere.' Dr. Playfair sees vivisection even where it does not exist. The marvel of Galvani's (or rather, I believe, the Signora Galvani's) discovery was, that it was possible to stimulate the muscles of *dead* frogs. Over that same balcony in Bologna now hangs the inscription commemorating that it was

DALLE MORTE RANE—

that Galvani *scoperse la Ellettricita animale*."—*Comments on the Debate in the House of Commons, April*, 1883, by Frances Power Cobbe (London, 1883), p. 16.

GELSEMIUM.—*See* YELLOW JASMINE.

GLAUCOMA, VON GRAEFE AND.   Bell Taylor.

CHARLES BELL TAYLOR, M.D.Edin., M.R.C.S.Eng., Hon.
Surgeon Nottingham and Midland Eye Infirmary. (A.V.)

"Von Graefe was led to the adoption of his method of
treatment by noticing that the excision of a piece of iris in his
men and women patients was followed by a marked diminution
of tension—in other words, a softening of the eyeball ; and as
increased tension or hardening of the eyeball constitutes the
essence of glaucoma, it is not to be wondered at that he
should have determined to try the effect of the same proceeding in cases of glaucoma. Von Graefe (whose practice I
have had the advantage of studying) assured me himself when
I was last in Berlin that his discovery was made in this way."
—*Letter in " Westminster Gazette,"* March 22nd, 1894, signed by
Charles Bell Taylor.

—— The same.   De Wecker.

L. DE WECKER, Professor of Clinical Ophthalmology, Medical
School, Paris. (P.V.)

"Von Graefe, having attended the clinique of the elder
Desmarres, had been struck by the remarkable results yielded
by paracentesis (*i.e.* tapping of the eyeball) in various
affections of the eye, and in glaucoma in particular. It did
not escape him how much more prolonged the relaxation was
in an eye, when the far more important paracentesis necessi-
tated by iridectomy (*i.e.* removal of a portion of the iris) had
been performed. It had been discovered that in glaucoma the
eye became very hard ; the means best suited to soften the eye
were resorted to, and the result was the happy discovery that
glaucoma might be cured by iridectomy."—*From the work on
" Ocular Therapeutics,"* by *L. de Wecker (translated by Dr.
Litton Forbes)* p. 269.

GUARANA.   Berdoe.

EDWARD BERDOE, M.R.C.S., L.R.C.P.Ed., London. (A.V.)

" Mantegazza, the inventor of a horrible machine for the
torture of small animals, which he called the ' Tormentatore,'
capable of inflicting graduated pain, termed by him according
to its degree ' intense,' ' cruel,' and ' most atrocious agony,'
experimented with guarana, and found that it excited frogs
and threw them into convulsions, that it influenced some

warm-blooded animals in a similar manner, but made rabbits dull and languid. and produced a sort of intoxication in dogs. 'It is curious,' says Stillé, 'to contrast these definite and striking results with those of Dr. Macdowall, of West Riding Insane Asylum. He experimented upon himself and two male attendants, and it soon became evident to him that even in very large doses its effect upon the body in a state of health is almost, if not quite, inappreciable.' Its action in fact is very similar to that of tea and coffee.'—*The Futility of Experiments with Drugs on Animals*, by Edward Berdoe (London, 1889), p. 23.

HARDENING EFFECTS.   Haughton.

REV. SAMUEL HAUGHTON, M.D., D.C.L., F.R.S., Proctor and Fellow of Trinity College, Dublin, a witness before the Royal Commission, 1875. (A.V.)

"My experience is that the dissecting room degrades some characters and elevates others; and knowing that it is a moral trial to any young man to pass through the ordeal of the hospital dead-house and the dissecting room, that it tries and tests his disposition, like the Lydian stone of the ancients, I would shrink with horror from accustoming large classes of young men to the sight of animals under vivisection. I believe that many of them would become cruel and hardened, and would go away and repeat these experiments recklessly, without foresight or forethought; science would gain nothing. and the world would have let loose upon it a set of young devils."—*Evidence Roy. Com.* (London, 1879), Q. 1,888.

—— The same.   Abernethy.

JOHN ABERNETHY (the late), F.R.S., Lecturer on Anatomy and Physiology, Royal College of Surgeons, London. (born 1764 : died 1831). (V.)

"The design of experiments is to interrogate nature; and surely the inquirer ought to make himself acquainted with the language of nature, and take care to propose pertinent questions; but I know that these experiments tend to harden the feelings, which often lead to the inconsiderate performance of them. Surely we should endeavour to foster, and not stifle benevolence, the best sentiment of our nature, that which is productive of the greatest gratification both to its possessor and to others. I, at the same time, express an earnest hope that the character of an English surgeon may never be tarnished by the commission of inconsiderate or unnecessary cruelty." —*Physiological Lectures*, No. iv.

HARDENING EFFECTS. Stephen.

LESLIE STEPHEN, Esq., Author, London. (R.)

" Many vivisectors are not medical men at all, and it has not yet become a proverb that physiologists are humane. The general tendency is obvious. Ordinary men are shocked at the sight of blood and torture. If they contemplate it frequently, the disgust ceases. A dissecting room turns a young student sick. In a few days he enters it as calmly as his study. In certain exceptional cases the instinctive delight passes into actual pleasure. It is a hideous but a notorious fact that cruelty is an actual source of delight to some boys and a few men. The fact might be illustrated from police reports, and even, it may be said in passing, by some modern literary developments. The mood which gloats over foul and cruel sights has been interpreted by artists of no small power, as well as in ' penny dreadfuls.' But this, we gladly admit, is an abnormal phenomenon. The surgeon learns to look at a wound with no sensation of physical disgust. If the disgust were not deadened, no man could be a surgeon.

❈   ❈   ❈   ❈   ❈

" Now, if we take the parallel case of vivisection, what is the ultimate end which causes a man to overlook the disagreeable means ? It is the promotion of science ; and science, it is added, is promoted with a view to the interests of humanity.

❈   ❈   ❈   ❈   ❈

" The medical student knows that the man of science has cut up a hundred cats to discover an infinitesimal fact. Why should not he cut up a single cat to verify an established fact ? His studies have familiarized him with the sight of blood and suffering, and he has therefore no instinctive repugnance to overcome. If he is a man of brutal nature, the disgust may even be replaced by a faint sense of pleasure. He regards his victim with a vague feeling of complacency or triumph."— *The Ethics of Vivisection, " Cornhill Magazine,"* April, 1886.

—— **The same.**—*See also* DEMORALISING EFFECTS *and* USE-LESSNESS (Johnson).

HEMLOCK LEAVES AND FRUIT (*Conium*), Berdoe.
Poison to Man, Harmless to Animals.

EDWARD BERDOE, M.R.C.S., L.R.C.P.Ed., London. (A.V.)

" Experimenters are much at variance as to the physiological action of conium. Some say that it slows the heart's action,

others deny this. Some declare that it increases the temperature of the body, others that it lowers it. One affirms that it
renders the blood dark and fluid, another protests that it has
no such effect. Summing up all these conflicting results, Dr.
Stillé says, 'These antagonistic results of experiments conducted under determinate conditions illustrate the difficulty of
drawing definite conclusions from such data and *the wisdom
of preferring clinical bases for clinical rules.'* (*National Dispensatory*, p. 456.)"—*The Futility of Experiments with Drugs on
Animals*, by Edward Berdoe (London, 1889), pp. 23, 24.

" Physiological experiments with this as with so many other
drugs already mentioned do not in the least help us to understand its actions when administered to human beings as a
medicine. From hemlock we obtain the alkaloid Conia. Guttman says this is one of the most active and powerful poisons
to human beings, being 'scarcely second to prussic acid.'
'Yet,' says Ringer, p. 437, 'some vegetable feeders, as the
goat, sheep, and horse, are said to eat hemlock with impunity.'
Can anything be more absurdly unscientific than to test on
these animals the action of a drug like hemlock for the discovery of its medical uses to man?"—*The Futility of Experiments with Drugs on Animals*, by Edward Berdoe (London,
1889). pp. 23, 24.

HENBANE LEAVES (*Hyoscyamus*).   Berdoe.

EDWARD BERDOE, M.R.C.S., L.R.C.P.Ed., London.   (A.V.)

" ' All parts of this plant are highly narcotic, and it is used in
medicine as a substitute for opium.' It is poisonous to fowls,
hence its name, henbane; yet on sheep, cows, and pigs it has
little or no effect. Hogs also can eat it with impunity."—
The Futility of Experiments with Drugs on Animals, by Edward
Berdoe (London, 1889), p. 24.

✝ HOSPITAL PATIENTS, The Use of.   de Watteville.

ARMAND DE WATTEVILLE, M.A., B.Sc., M.D.Bale, M.R.C.S.
   Eng., Physician West End Hospital for Nervous Diseases, London.
   (V.)

" A few days ago an anonymous letter appeared in your
columns which, emanating (as the signature ' M.D.' appeared to
show) from a medical practitioner, ought not to be allowed to
pass without an energetic protest.

" As far as I can see, the writer intends to bring a charge
against a distinguished member of his own profession—a
physician who by his labours in the field of therapeutics has

done eminent service to medicine, and has been instrumental
to the relief of much human suffering—a serious charge, I say,
viz. that of having used patients in a hospital for other purposes than those tending to their own direct benefit.

"Now, I should like to ask 'M.D.' whether his whole career
as a medical student, from the day he handled his first bone to
that on which he passed his last clinical examination, did not
involve abuses very similar to those for which he now joins the
unfortunately ever-growing pseudo-humanitarian outcry against
the methods of rational medicine?

"What right had he to trample upon the feelings of others in
dissecting the bodies of people whose sole crime was to have
been poor, and, still more, to acquire his clinical experience at
the expense of, perhaps, much human shame and suffering?

"I think we, as medical men, should not attempt to conceal
from the public the debt of gratitude they owe to the ' corpora
vilia '—for such there are, and will be, as long as the healing
art exists and progresses. So far from there being a reason
why moral and pecuniary support should be refused to hospitals
on the ground that their inmates are made use of otherwise than for treatment, there is even ground why more
and more should be given to them, in order to compensate by
every possible comfort for the discomforts necessarily entailed
by the education of succeeding generations of medical men,
and the improvements in our methods of coping with disease.

"No amount of hysterical agitation and so-called humani
tarian agitation will alter the laws of Nature, one of the plainest
of which is that the few must suffer for the many. Sentimentalists who think they know better, who uphold the abstract
' Rights of Man,' and want to push them to their logical consequences, have no other alternative in the question now before
us than to condemn the modern course of medical studies, and
trust themselves into the hands of bookmen, whose *tactus
eruditus* will then have to be formed at their expense. The
fundamental question at issue is not whether in this or that
instance improper use was made of a hospital patient, but
whether the manipulations and observations indispensable for
the acquisition and extension of medical knowledge are to be
made in a connected and enlightened manner, in public institu-
tions, and under the eyes of experienced men, or to be left to
the isolated, haphazard, and groping efforts of necessarily
ignorant men upon the persons of any who may be found to
pay them in the hope of benefiting by their medical skill.

"Whilst defending the moral grounds upon which experimental medicine rests, I allow that there are limits, narrow

limits, beyond which it would be imprudent or criminal to go.
But I must emphatically protest against the tendency of men
nowadays—and I am ashamed to observe that a few are to be
found within the medical profession itself—who act upon the
supposition that the public at large form a proper tribunal to
decide upon what constitutes a transgression of those limits.
Those alone are competent judges who are able to form
a correct opinion on the one hand of the ultimate utility, on
the other of the proximate consequences, of any investigation
in corpore vili."—*Letter in the* " *Standard,*" November 24th, 1883.

HUMAN BEINGS, Experiments on.   Celsus.

AURELIUS CORNELIUS CELSUS, Roman Physician and
Philosopher of the Augustan age. (A.V.)

" Celsus, in Book III., on noticing the dissection of
criminals, says :—' It is unprofitable and cruel *to lay open* with
the knife living bodies, so that the art which is designed for
the protection and relief of suffering is made to inflict injury,
and that of the most atrocious nature. If in the entire and
uninjured body we can often, by external observation, perceive
remarkable changes produced from fear, pain, hunger,
weariness, and a thousand other affections, how much
greater must be changes induced by the dreadful wounds and
cruel manglings of the dissector in internal parts, whose
structure is far more delicate, and which are placed in
circumstances altogether unusual.' These unanswerable
observations increase in power and aptness when applied
to the lower creatures, because, if vivisections were profitless,
misleading, cruel, and atrocious, as depicted by Celsus when
the dissections were performed on men and women, creatures
of the race to be benefited, the experiments are doubly false
when inflicted upon animals of totally different species."—
Dr. Bowie's Reply to Dr. Rutherford, 24th Dec., 1880 (*Review*
Office, 20, St. Giles' Street, Edinburgh), p. 5.

—— The same.   Lister.

SIR JOSEPH LISTER, Bart., F.R.S., Emeritus Professor of Clinical
Surgery in King's College, London. (V.)

" I have not yet ventured to make the experiment on any large
scale, though I have long had it in contemplation. It is a
serious thing to experiment upon the lives of our fellow-men,
but I believe the time has now arrived when it may be tried."—
*Address before the International Medical Congress at Berlin,
reported in the* " *British Medical Journal,*" Aug. 16th, 1890,
p. 379.

HUMAN BEINGS.—Experiments on,   Macaulay,

JAMES MACAULAY, M.A., M.D., F.R.C.S.Ed., London.   (A.V.)

" There is another way of looking at the question of vivi-section, as tending to human benefit. If it is right to perform experiments on living bodies for advancement of the healing art, why not perform them on human bodies ? It has been done in past times, and may be proposed again. If condemned malefactors were operated upon, it would only be anticipating, by a brief period, their hour of death. Or the experiments might be made on the insane and imbecile, or persons defective in intellectual or moral faculties, but with animal life in natural vigour. The subjects would be free from the objections arising out of the different structure, constitution, and functions of the lower animals, though still liable to certain fallacies inseparable from the very method of research. Vivisectors make light of these alleged fallacies, and think their experiments full of light and fruit. Fair argument might be used for experiments on living men, with or without anæsthetics, as the inquiry might demand. It might be argued that it is expedient or right that one or a few should suffer for the benefit of the human family. And if the argument, ' *in majus bonum*,' were strengthened by reference to *corpora vilia*, then of malefactors doomed to die, and of imbeciles, this could be truly said."—*Vivisection : A Prize Essay* (London, 1881), p. 76.

—— The same.   Murrell and Ringer.

WILLIAM MURRELL, M.D., M.R.C.S., Lecturer on Materia Medica and Therapeutics, Westminster Hospital, London (V.) : and SYDNEY RINGER, M.D., F.R.C.P., Holme Professor of Clinical Medicine, University College, London. (V.)

" In addition to these experiments, we have made some observations clinically. To eighteen adults—fourteen men and four women—we ordered ten grains of the pure nitrite of sodium in an ounce of water, and of these seventeen declared that they were unable to take it. . . . One man, a burly, strong fellow, suffering from a little rheumatism only, said that after taking the first dose he ' felt giddy,' as if he would ' go off insensible.' His lips, face, and hands turned blue, and he had to lie down for an hour and a half before he dared move. His heart fluttered, and he suffered from throbbing pains in the head. He was urged to take another dose, but declined on the ground that he had a wife and family. Another patient had to sit down for an hour after the dose, and said that it

' took all his strength away.' He, too, seemed to think that the medicine did not agree with him. . . . The women appear to have suffered more than the men. . . . One woman said that ten minutes after taking the first dose—she did not try a second—she felt a trembling sensation all over her, and suddenly fell on the floor. Whilst lying there she perspired profusely, her face and head seemed swollen and throbbed violently, until she thought they would burst. . . . Another woman said she thought she would have died after taking a dose; it threw her into a violent perspiration, and in less than five minutes her lips turned quite black and throbbed for hours; it upset her so much that she was afraid she would never get over it. The only one of the fourteen patients who made no complaint after taking ten grains was powerfully affected by fifteen. . . . The effect on these patients was so unpleasant that it was deemed unadvisable to increase the dose."—*Drs. Ringer and Murrell in "The Lancet,"* Nov. 3rd, 1883.

HUMAN BEINGS—Epitome of Published   Thornhill. Accounts of Experiments on,

MARK THORNHILL, Esq., Ex-Indian Judge, Author of "*Experiments on Hospital Patients,*" etc., Dover. (A.V.)

A.

" Experiment with ' Curare ' on two children at Manchester. —*Evid. Roy. Com.* (London, 1876), Q. 5,407.

" Experiments on varnishing the skin—so frequently tried on animals—tried on men.—*British Medical Journal*, May 11th, 1878, p. 671.

" Patients admitted to hospital in dying condition, made the subject of minute and tedious examinations, merely to furnish reports to the medical journals.—*British Medical Journal*, June 7th, 1879.

" Experiment of producing convulsions in a woman by tickling and pricking her feet.—*British Medical Journal*, March 25th, 1882.

" Patient admitted to a hospital suffering from a most painful skin disease; ' he was in a most miserable condition from pain and irritation.' His cure was purposely delayed, in order to demonstrate to the students that nature alone, without treatment, would not effect it.—*British Medical Journal*, January 7th, 1882, p. 5.

" Experiment of producing acute gout by administration of salts of lead.—*Ringer's Handbook of Therapeutics*, p. 256.

K

" Poor woman, admitted to hospital in a dying condition, made the subject of constant observation and examination with tuning forks, etc. These examinations were continued till her death, which occurred twenty-four hours after her admission.—*British Medical Journal*, October 27th, 1883.

" Experiment of injecting milk into the veins of a dying patient.—*British Medical Journal*, June 6th, 1885.

"Variety of experiments on hospital patients with drugs. The medical man who performed these experiments states explicitly that they were such, 'and had no bearing on disease.' —*British Medical Journal*, November 28th, 1885, pp. 1005 and 1011.

" Experiment of producing a hideous disease by inoculation with the matter from sores of persons suffering from it.'— *British Medical Journal*, January 9th, 1886, p. 57.

" Calabar bean having been found to produce epileptic fits in rabbits, its effects were tried with similar results on human beings.—*Wood's Therapeutics*, p. 319.

" Mr. Stanford Harris states that in one medical work alone—Dr. Ringer's *Handbook of Therapeutics*—experiments are described performed on patients by no less than nine different surgeons and physicians as to the effects of drugs,* the drugs in all the cases being administered for the pure purpose of experiment, and having no relation to the maladies of the patients. The administration of the drugs produced painful, in some instances dangerous, effects.

" I quote from Mr. Harris's pamphlet the following instances: The drug gelseminum is a powerful paralyser and respiratory poisoner. It is described as having been administered to six persons on seventeen occasions, in order merely to ascertain its effects on human beings. In the course of this series of experiments, the drug was administered in doses sufficiently large to produce ' toxic ' (poisonous) effects.

" It was also administered on thirty-three occasions to test its effect on the circulation. On these occasions the full ' toxic ' (poisonous) effects were produced. The effects are described as ' giddiness,' ' dimness of sight,' ' strong double internal squint,' ' weakness of the legs,' ' severe headache,' and ' dull aching pain in the eyeballs.'

" The effects of the drug ' salicine ' were similarly studied on human subjects—patients in the hospitals. The patients selected for the experiments were ' healthy children,' ' to whom doses were given sufficient to produce ' toxic ' (poisonous) effects.' The results were ' headaches, often so severe that the

---

* *Vivisection and the Treatment of Patients*, p. 1.

patient buries his head in his pillow: ' ' muscular weakness and tremors,' ' slight fever,' etc.; ' twitchings and tremblings of the legs and arms.'

" The first set of experiments with this drug were made, it is said, on a boy of ten. He had been admitted into the hospital with ' belladonna poisoning.' But, it is stated, ' the observations were not commenced till some days after his complete recovery.' The effects produced on this child by the drug were ' severe frontal headache,' so severe ' that the lad shut his eyes, buried his head in his pillow, and, though a lively boy, became very dull and stupid. He complained of a tingling like pins and needles in his right ankle, and suffered from very decided muscular weakness, soon accompanied by muscular twitchings and tremblings of the legs and arms.'

" Another boy—it is stated that the symptoms continued so long after the administration of the last dose that the experimenters ' became alarmed.' ' They did not know how long or to what degree they (the symptoms) might increase.' ' Sixty-five hours after the last dose he (the boy) was still dull, rather deaf, and there was a slight tremor of the hands.'—*Vivisection and Treatment of Patients*, pp. 6 to 9.

" In the work above referred to—*Handbook of Therapeutics*, by Dr. Ringer—some experiments on the effect of alcohol on the temperature of the human body are described, and others referred to. These experiments appear to have been performed on numerous patients on several occasions by at least five English physicians, and on persons of all ages, some being children. The alcohol in some of the cases, it is recorded, was administered ' in poisonous ' doses. ' On one boy, aged ten, a large number of observations were made.' One man, mentioned as an ' habitual drunkard,' was dosed with alcohol till he was made ' dead drunk.'

" To one ' healthy young man ' two physicians administered for six days a daily amount of absolute alcohol, varying from one to six ounces.' On a subsequent occasion they administered to him ' twelve ounces of brandy daily for a period of three days.'—*Handbook of Therapeutics*, pp. 342 and 343, 11th edition.

" *Note.*—Some of these experiments appear to have been supplementary to some similar experiments on rabbits, as a comparison is made between the effects of the alcohol on the temperature in rabbits and in human beings."

B.

" Dr. Wachsmuth performed a series of experiments on his

own son, which he himself describes. The child suffered from hæmorrhagic diathesis. Dr. Wachsmuth ascertained that the attacks of the disease, when they came on, could be cured by a certain medicine. and that when they threatened they could be prevented by another medicine. But having made this discovery, Dr. Wachsmuth did not avail himself of it. He allowed the child to remain without treatment that he might study the development of the disease. I have quoted from Mr. Stanford Harris's pamphlet, p. 10 ; the case is mentioned in *Holme's System of Surgery*, 2nd edition, vol. i. p. 722.

" Dr. Lund, of the Island of Samsö, in Denmark, also performed a series of experiments on his own child. They are described in vol. xi. of the *Scandinavian Medical Archives*, 1879, in an article by Dr. Salomon on inoculation of tuberculosis, in the following words :—' Many experiments have been made in the last few years by administering the flesh and milk of tuberculous cattle to animals. The Danish physician, Dr. Lund, of the Isle of Samsö, communicated the particulars of an experiment on a human being. The milk was taken from a wretched, meagre cow, continually coughing and suffering from inflammation of the lungs. The subject of the experiment was Dr. Lund's youngest son, a healthy, well-made boy. The baby was fed with milk from the said cow from February, 1865, to November of the same year ; and from November, 1865, to August, 1867, the child was fed with the milk of another similar cow.' The result of the experiment is described as follows :—' When eight months old, scrofulous conjunctivitis appeared in the child, which still continued when Dr. Lund wrote his report. In Dr. Lund's opinion the disease could only be rationally accounted for by reference to the diseased milk.' —*Zoophilist*, April, 1884, p. 284.

" Experiment of Bargigli on two children. Aug. Hirsch in his *Handbuch der Historisch geographischen Pathologie*, 2nd Abtheilung, 1883, p. 32, speaks of the criminal experiment made by Bargigli in inoculating children, from six to eight years old, with the matter of a leprous tumour. Hirsch quotes Bargigli's own words. The *Zoophilist*, after quoting the description, adds, ' Thus it appears that hapless children of six and eight years old were sold by their parents or guardians to Bargigli, to risk death by leprosy merely to satisfy that man of science of the truth or falsehood of his theory on the nature of that hideous disease."—*Zoophilist*, April, 1884, p. 284.

" Experiment on children. Dr. Stickles, of Paris, inoculated twelve children with the nasal discharge from four rabbits and a dog who had been inoculated with the same discharge from a horse, who was suffering from a disease to which horses are subject, resembling scarlet fever. The children became ill, an eruption came out. their glands swelled, their skin peeled. After this they were inoculated with the blood of persons suffering from scarlatina, and did not take the disease. Quoted by New York *Medical Times* of August, 1888, from *Gazette Médicale de Paris.*—*Zoophilist*, September, 1888, pp. 79, 80.

" It is stated on the authority of M. Victor Meunier that a Dr. Pellican endeavoured to produce spontaneous combustion in women who were confirmed drunkards. ' When they were nearly insensible with drink, he plied them with as much spirits as they could swallow. and then applied a lighted match to their mouths.'—*Zoophilist.* January, 1888, p. 147.

" Experiments on Mary Rafferty. These experiments were performed at the Good Samaritan Hospital, at Cincinnati. in America. Mary Rafferty was a servant maid. She was admitted into the hospital suffering from some disease or accident, in consequence of which portions of her skull had become removed, leaving the brain exposed. Her recovery appeared hopeless, and the surgeon or physician attending her considered himself justified in making her the subject of experiments on the functions of the brain. In the course of these experiments needles were thrust through the dura mater into the substance of the brain. The brain was then stimulated by galvanic or electric shocks. The agony of these experiments must have been extreme. Mary Rafferty died, it is said, in consequence of these experiments. I think she died during their performance. The experiments are said to have been undertaken as supplemental to those performed in England by Dr. Ferrier on cats and monkeys." Mr. Thornhill adds : " The full details of these experiments are given, I believe, in the *British Medical Journal* of 22nd May, 1874. They are referred to in the evidence taken before the Royal Commission on Vivisection in 1875, Q. 3,390, and it is there stated that the experiments were believed to have caused the death of the patient. I have taken the above account from the *Zoophilist* of December, 1883."

" Experiment on the Italian Rinalducci. This experiment was performed by Dr. Ezio Sciamanna, and described by himself in a paper on the ' Phenomena produced by the Application of the Electric Current to the Dura Mater.' The object of the experiment, it is stated, was to ascertain whether excitation of the brain produces in man the same results as in apes. Rinalducci was admitted into the hospital at Turin on March 23rd, 1882, suffering from fracture of the skull. He underwent the operation of trepanning, which left a portion of the surface of the brain exposed. His recovery appearing hopeless, as in the case of Mary Rafferty, he was made the subject of experiment. The details of the experiment are thus described:—A galvanic battery having been brought, the 'negative electrode was moved over the surface of the brain, and notes taken of the motor phenomena. The intensity of the current was felt to the ends of the fingers. The patient was not asleep. Choral anæsthesia was only once attempted, and then ineffectually.' The results of the experiment were as follow :—' The mouth of the patient closed, each jaw being in tetanic contraction. Movements took place of the arm and left hand, and rotation of the head to the left, opening of the mouth, etc. On dissection after death the exact points of the brain were perceived which had been excited,' the brain, I presume, having been burnt, or inflamed, by the passage of the galvanic current.—From the *Zoophilist* of December, 1883, pp. 310-313.

"*Note*.—In order that the intensity of agony that these experiments must have caused may be understood, I add an account of the behaviour of animals when undergoing similar and even less severe operations. In these cases the ordinary conditions were reversed. The animals being in health could by their screams and movements express their sufferings—the human subjects of the experiments were unable to do so. In Dr. Ferrier's experiments, which were identical with those performed on Mary Rafferty and Rinalducci, the behaviour of a cat when its brain was being similarly stimulated by galvanic shocks is thus described:—The animal screamed, kicked out with its left hind leg, gnawed its own legs, panted, screamed, as if in furious rage, uttered long-continued cries.—*Evidence, Royal Commission Report* (London, 1876), pp. 220–221.

" The animals in a menagerie in America were subjected lately to mere ordinary galvanic shocks. The shocks were of extreme power, but were administered merely to the limbs or body, not to the exposed brain. These were the results :—A baboon ' became wild with rage,' other animals ' seemed paralysed,' the monkeys ' screamed and seemed to be undergoing agonies,' a wolf ' cried piteously.' One dog had only a moderate current of electricity passed through the base of the brain, but the effect was such that he became mad within half an hour, and had to be killed.—From the *Zoophilist* of March, 1889, p. 206.

" The following experiment was performed by three medical men at Syra, in Greece. It was reported in the *British Medical Journal* of June 17th, 1882, p. 897, in a lecture given by Dr. B.

Yeo. The lecturer is not represented as having expressed any disapproval of the experiment:—

"A man whose lungs were perfectly healthy was suffering from a gangrene in his foot. His death appearing inevitable, it was thought justifiable to inoculate him, by way of experiment, with the 'sputum' and blood of a woman suffering from consumption. Three weeks after the inoculation tubercles appeared in the lungs. In thirty-eight days the man died.—From the *Zoophilist* of June, 1884. The experiment is described in greater detail in '*Dying Scientifically*' (London, 1888), pp. 113–116.

"In the *Medical Press* of December 5th, 1888, p. 583, is an account of an experiment performed by a foreign physician on one of his patients, a poor woman. She was suffering from cancer in the left breast. By way of experiment, pieces of the cancerous skin were cut off, and engrafted on to the healthy skin of the right breast; the cancer was, in consequence, there also developed.—The woman is said to have died from this extension of the disease.—From the *Zoophilist* of January, 1889, pp. 154 and 155.

"The *Dublin Medical Journal* of September, 1885, p. 153, describes an experiment made in Italy on the exposed brain of a patient who had lost a portion of his skull. The experiment was made with drugs.—From *Zoophilist* of October, 1888, p. 95.

"The *British Medical Journal* describes a series of experiments performed abroad—in Paris, by Fehling, on infants, with various drugs. The drugs were given to the women who were nursing the children, and the effect on the infants noted. The drugs were of the most deleterious, even poisonous, character, consisting of salicylate of soda, iodide of potassium, ferro-cyanide of potassium, iodoform, mercury, morphia, chloral, atropine, and others.—*Dying Scientifically* (London, 1888), pp. 86–7."

HUMAN BEINGS—DEMAND FOR MORE   Pyle.
EXPERIMENTS ON.

J. S. PYLE, M.D., American Physician. (P.V.)

"It is certain that experimental work upon the seats of human consciousness will assist us materially in an exposition of the subject. No other method of study or investigation will ever penetrate the secret regions of cerebral action and disclose the capacity and functional limits of the phosphorised proteid matter constituting the cerebral nerve cells. Under the influence of stimulus, in the form of a mild electric current, the cells can be made to repeat their official work and reproduce in consciousness the direct result of their operations. . . . It is plain, if we are to make any great headway in such investigation, our inquiry must be addressed to consciousness. The ego must be interrogated and made to locate the operations of all its integral parts. The stimulus will have to be applied when the individual subjected to the examination is in a perfectly lucid state of mind, and an application need not be the least unpleasant. To secure co-operation and carry out the experiment successfully the condemned would be instructed with the nature of the work, assured that no torture would be instituted; that the preparation of removing a piece of the skull and cerebral membranes should take place when under the influence of an anæsthetic; and, while he would be allowed to regain consciousness to be interrogated, that no pain would be occasioned thereby; lastly, that his death should occur when in a profound sleep. This would, it would seem, remove the appearance of revenge and barbarity, and convert such an occasion into one of real utility, both socially and scientifically."—*Dr. J. S. Pyle, in the "American Journal of Politics,"* December, 1893.

HYDROGEN, Peroxide of.   Berdoe.

EDWARD BERDOE, M.R.C.S., L.R.C.P.Ed., London.   (A.V.)

" Many experiments have been made upon rabbits and dogs by injecting this gas under their skin; it caused severe obstruction to the breathing, then convulsions and death. But Guttman injected a solution of the gas into one side of a rabbit's abdomen, and a solution of sulphate of iron into the other, and found that the animal did not die. The experimenters thought they had discovered something useful to humanity by these experiments. 'But,' says Stillé, 'though upon theoretical grounds this compound was introduced as a cure for *diabetes,* it signally failed after a sufficient trial by competent judges.'— (*National Dispensatory*, p. 746) "—*The Futility of Experiments with Drugs on Animals,* by Edward Berdoe (London, 1889), p. 25.

HYDROPHOBIA—M. Pasteur and Lord Doneraile's Case.

M. PASTEUR'S STATEMENT.—" Professor Grancher and Dr. Roux yielded to the desire which was so warmly expressed; several inoculations were practised, but without using medullæ of more [strength] than five days' drying. Carried out under such conditions, the treatment could only, alas! delay the de-velopment of the rabic virus for four or five months."--*Letter signed "L. Pasteur," in the "British Medical Journal,"* Sept. 17th, 1887.

LADY DONERAILE'S REJOINDER.—"We are informed that several of M. Pasteur's statements in his letter to the *British Medical Journal.* on the subject of Lord Doneraile's death from hydrophobia, are not correct. and the family considers them very unfair. Lady Doneraile never urged him not to try what was called the 'intensive' process; but as a person was supposed to have just died from the effects of it at the time that the fox bit Lord Doneraile, he himself naturally objected to running the risk of being killed by that avowedly not yet fully under-stood form of the treatment. He was, moreover, told by both Professor Grancher and Dr. Roux that the original (not 'in-tensive') inoculations were perfectly efficacious; and he was certainly not told that it, as M. Pasteur now for the credit of his discovery affirms, would keep off hydrophobia for only four or five months! Moreover, it was said by every one connected with the *Institut Pasteur* that people would be preserved from hydrophobia if treated by the Pasteur system within thirty days from the time of being bitten, and Lord Doneraile's treatment was begun within twelve days."—*Cork Constitution*, Oct. 18th, 1887.

HYDROPHOBIA—Pasteur and Jenner. Kingsford.

ANNA KINGSFORD, M.D., Paris (the late). (A.V.)

" Pasteur's system differs radically from that of Jenner. The latter represents an attempt to guarantee the economy against a certain malady by the artificial introduction of the virus of an analogous but far milder malady, characteristic of the bovine race, and having the property, it is asserted, of diminishing in the human race the natural susceptibility to variola. This vac-cine, being a special and distinct substance, having a special and distinct nature, is procurable directly and without further preparation from the tissues of any child or adult recently in-oculated with it. But the 'attenuated virus' of M. Pasteur's school is quite another thing. It is in no sense a 'vaccine,' it does not represent a special and natural disease, but a manu-factured disease, a substance artificially prepared, and of which the efficacy is so rapidly destructible that it is necessary to pro-duce it afresh from week to week."—" *Recent Researches in Hydrophobia,*" " *Illustrated Science Monthly,*" August, 1884.

HYDROPHOBIA.   Bell Taylor.

CHARLES BELL TAYLOR, M.D.Edin., M.R.C.S.Eng., Hon.
Surgeon Nottingham and Midlan l Eye Infirmary.   (A.Y.)

" By vaccination we give the patient something which is considered equivalent to small pox in a mild form, and so place him
in the position of one who has had the disease ; and if there
was the slightest reason for supposing that hydrophobia was a
disease of this kind—if rabies in the dog was the same disease
as hydrophobia in the man—if the patient were inoculated before being bitten—if there was the slightest ground for concluding that a patient who had had hydrophobia once could not
have it again (which there is not), and if M. Pasteur by his
inoculations could cause hydrophobia in a mild form, and so
protect his patients against a fatal attack,—then the comparison which is so often made between his injections and Jenner's
system of vaccination would hold good. But M. Pasteur's
injections produce no effect whatever unless they cause hydrophobia, and when they do cause hydrophobia the patient usually
dies. If we vaccinate a patient who has not been vaccinated
before, and the vaccination does not take—if no constitutional
disturbance results—if there be no rise of temperature, no swelling, no redness, no pain, no formation of vesicles containing
inoculable lymph,—then the patient is certainly not protected,
but is in precisely the same condition as one who has not
been vaccinated at all; and if we subject a patient who has
been bitten by a mad dog to a series of hypodermic injections
that produce no effect whatever, no constitutional disturbance,
no fever, no hydrophobic symptoms, no local irritation, then he
is clearly just as likely to die of hydrophobia as he would be
if nothing had been done."—*Pasteur's Prophylactic, from the
" National Review*," July, 1890.

—— The same—Pasteur's Method : Proof   Richards.
of Patients' Danger Wanting.

VINCENT RICHARDS (the late), M.R.C.S.Edin., M.R.C.S.Eng.,
Goalundo, Bengal. (V.)

" I do not propose here entering into a discussion of the
merits of M. Pasteur's method; but I cannot help saying that
there appears to exist an unreasoning acceptance of assertions
in its favour to the exclusion of facts which are unfavourable.
So far as I can gather, the very essentials of proof on scientific
grounds are wanting. There is nothing whatever to show that
the numerous persons being inoculated at his laboratory were
bitten by rabid animals, if we except the fatal cases ; nor is

there anything to show how far immunity from rabies may have been due to causes other than those claimed by M. Pasteur."—*Letter in " The Lancet,"* June 26th, 1886.

HYDROPHOBIA—M. Pasteur and.   Colin.

M. COLIN, Professor at the French Veterinary School, at Alfort. (V.)

"You say there have been about 2,400 persons bitten ; we will allow that, but that they were all bitten by mad dogs is more than improbable. The certificates produced by the patients are worth nothing ; they were drawn up by incompetent people, and cannot be verified. The *post mortem* examinations of the dogs are equally valueless ; they afford no evidence of the madness of the dogs. The only way of arriving at a certain conclusion is by the prolonged observation of the animal, which should be shut up and kept till the characteristic symptoms declare themselves. It is therefore evident that a great number of the persons reputed to be under the influence of hydrophobia were bitten by dogs that were never mad at all."—*Speech before the French Academy of Medicine*, Paris, Nov. 9th, 1886.

—— The same—Bite of Healthy Dog   Pasteur.
   will not produce.

LOUIS PASTEUR, Director of the Pasteur Institute, Paris. (V.)

" M. Pasteur has had pleasure in receiving your letter of the 31st of May. The bite of a dog is only dangerous when the dog has got rabies. If there is any doubt in respect to this, the manner in which it may be found out is the following :—Put the dog that has bitten where it can do no further harm. Have it examined by a vet., and if it has the rabies its characteristic symptoms will not be long before they are observed, and the animal will certainly die in eight days. If at the end of that time no symptoms of rabies has been observed, the bite cannot cause hydrophobia, and there is no reason that the animal should be destroyed."—*Letter signed " F. Menu," addressed to Miss Alicia Flint, The Priory, Newhaven Road, Edinburgh, and published in the " Scotsman,"* November 6th, 1894.

—— The same—Pasteur's System   Fleming.
   perpetuates Hydrophobia.

GEORGE FLEMING, M.R.C.V.S., formerly Veterinary Inspector-General to the Army. (P.V.)

" I have said nothing as to the preventive, or rather protective, treatment of rabies and hydrophobia introduced by M. Pasteur, for the reason that when we might suppress the disease altogether in this country, it would seem worse than foolish to keep it always with us—with its terrors, risks and inconveniences—and have to, at the same time, either send bitten persons (we could not well send animals) to Paris to be protectively inoculated, or to provide one or more expensive establishments on this side of the Channel for this purpose, in which rabbits must be dying from the disorder every day all the year round, in order that their spinal cords might be prepared for inoculating some chance person who had been wounded by a mad or suspected dog. Such a procedure would not look very sensible, or even humane, so far as the rabbits were concerned at least."—*Nineteenth Century*, March, 1890.

HYDROPHOBIA—Pasteur's Limitations. Bell.

ERNEST BELL, M.A., London. (A.V.)

"Will you allow me to state a few reasons for doubting whether the percentage of deaths which Pasteur chronicles is any proof of the efficacy of his treatment? At first he told us positively that his method would protect all patients at any time before hydrophobia actually broke out, but since then he has introduced many limitations; for—

"1. He does not now profess to protect unless the patient comes to him within a fortnight of being bitten.

"2. He does not reckon deaths which occur during the treatment.

"3. He does not recognise those which occur within a fortnight after the end of the treatment.

"4. He does not attempt to keep any record of his patients after that time.

"5. He does not even include in his lists deaths which occur afterwards, and are duly chronicled elsewhere.

"6. He does not claim that his inoculations have permanent effect. Re-inoculation, he says, is necessary after a time.

"7. He does not hesitate to swell his successes by any number of patients who were never in any danger of contracting the disease.

"8. He does not mind adding to his total cases which infringe one or all of these conditions, *provided they do not die.*

"9. He does not know how his so-called protective inoculations act.

"10. He does not know what is the cause of rabies.

"There is really hardly a loophole left by which the most

malevolent patient could die if he wished ever so much to do so, and for these limitations there is no scientific ground whatever."—*Letter in the " St. James's Gazette" (London)*, May 1st, 1894.

HYDROPHOBIA—Unreliability of   Dowdeswell.
Pasteur's Inferences.

GEORGE FRANCIS DOWDESWELL, M.A., F.C.S., F.R.S., (the late), London. (V.)

" Lastly, [it was found] that with respect to the methods of protection against infection by a series of inoculations with modified virus, as advocated and practised by M. Pasteur, these are unsuccessful with the rabbit, and that his recent ' rapid' or 'intensive' method of inoculation is liable itself to produce infection ; and that with the dog, the natural refractoriness of this animal to infection with rabies with any method of inoculation is so great that it is exceedingly difficult to determine the effect of any remedial or prophylactic measure upon it : and that with man the statistics of the treatment must determine its results."—*From a Paper read before the Royal Society*, June 18th, 1887.

—— The same—The Deaths after   Dolan.
M. Pasteur's Treatment.

THOMAS M. DOLAN, M.D., Author of " Rabies or Hydrophobia " (London, 1879), Horton House, Halifax. (R.)

" We need not expect M. Pasteur's experiments to form an opinion on the merits of his method ; time has solved part of the question. The deaths after his preventive inoculation are the saddest corollaries we could have on the falseness of the basis on which his prophylactic rested.

      ❊   ❊   ❊   ❊   ❊

" M. Pasteur has had numerous deaths, and now we are assured that it is a question of averages. He has had better results than any other hydrophobia curer. The ground has been so repeatedly shifted, that there is a great difficulty in dealing with M. Pasteur."—*Letter signed " T. M. Dolan, M.D.," in " British Medical Journal,"* Sept. 4th, 1886.

—— The same—M. Pasteur's Rabbit Rabies.   Dolan.

THOMAS M. DOLAN, M.D., Author of " Rabies or Hydrophobia " (London, 1879), Horton House, Halifax. (R.)

" M. Pasteur produced a disease in rabbits which he called

rabies. The same kind of affection in rabbits can be produced by injecting almost any kind of diseased material into the same region favoured by M. Pasteur. In man, the symptoms of hydrophobia can be also produced by irritating the medulla ; and in certain states we find a disease simulating hydrophobia, produced by a tumour or by cysticerci pressing on the brain. (See *Practitioner*, 1881, for a case narrated by the writer.)"— *Letter signed " T. M. Dolan, M.D.," in " British Medical Journal,"* Sept. 4th, 1886.

HYDROPHOBIA—Dangers of Inoculation   James.
of Intensive Virus.

CONSTANTIN JAMES, M.D. (the late), of Paris ; a former pupil of Majendie. (V.)

" As for the inoculation, and especially the *intensive* inoculation, I confess that it inspires me with a repugnance that nearly amounts to terror.   For, in short, supposing myself to be the bitten person, how should I go to have inoculated in my veins 'torrents' of the very same virus that I had taken all possible pains to destroy to the remotest particle by cauterisation ?   Besides, it seems to me that my imagination would remain continually haunted by the hydrophobia spectre which would perpetually remind me that there was no prescription available against that malady so long as the germ remained." —*Le Moniteur Universel*, Paris, Feb., 1887.

—— The same—The Truth about   Dolan.
Pasteur's Vaccine.

THOMAS M. DOLAN, M.D., Author of " Rabies or Hydrophobia " (London, 1879), Horton House, Halifax. (R.)

" M. Pasteur has treated a large number of persons bitten by non-rabid dogs. He has also treated a number who were not even bitten, but who had been licked by dogs. He has even injected with his *bouillon* persons never bitten, but who submitted to the process through curiosity. He has ventured to treat these persons with a virus, said to be even more potent than the virus of the rabid stray dog. No ill results have followed, not even an abscess, only a slight erythematous redness at the end of the inoculations. This is not only strange, but it even reduces the value of his virus to an absurdity. If the virus had protective virtues, it should have manifested itself in some way. If the virus were injected, so as to counteract in any way another virus already in the system, then it would be of no use in the case of those persons bitten by non-rabid dogs, or in the case of those not bitten by a dog. Yet we are assured, in the face of such manifest objections, that M. Pasteur continues his injections, and exposes all these persons to the danger of a virus, so intense as to rival that of the wandering rabid dog. What is the explanation? M. Pasteur has been injecting all this time a *sterilised bouillon*. Hence the safety of his patients; and I may say it is fortunate for his patients that he has been so doing. I shall be answered that he tested the virus on rabbits. I answer yes, but not by simple inoculation into the skin, but into the rabbits' medulla; and were he to do the same with the human subject, he would infallibly kill his patients, who would die with symptoms of hydrophobia."—*Letter of T. M. Dolan, M.D., " British Medical Journal*," Sept. 4th, 1886.

HYDROPHOBIA--Average Mortality of Persons Bitten.   Horsley.

VICTOR HORSLEY, F.R.C.S., M.B., F.R.S., Professor of Pathology, University College, London. (V.)

June 27th, 1887.—"After the first few months in which M. Pasteur practised his treatment, he was occasionally obliged, in order to quiet fears, to inoculate persons who believed that they had been bitten by rabid animals, but could give no satisfactory evidence of it. It might, therefore, be deemed unjust to estimate the total value of his treatment in the whole of his cases as being more than is represented by the difference between the rate of mortality observed in them and the lowest rate observed in any large number of cases not inoculated. This lowest rate may be taken at 5 per cent."—*Report of Local Government Board Committee*, pp. iv. v.

June 28th, 1887.—"What percentage of persons bitten by rabid dogs escape? The records upon that point are very various; they have been stated very highly by some, and very low by others. The lowest records state that 5 per cent. die; that rests only on a very small number of cases. The most usual record that has been accepted is 15 per cent., but I fancy the general belief of most of us would be that it is about 10 per cent."—*Minutes of Evidence, Lords Committee on Rabies*, 1887, Q. 215.

Feb. 12th, 1889.—"We are concerned with but one death-rate,—namely, that of groups of persons bitten by rabid dogs, the rabidity being established by the fact of one or more individuals of the group dying of rabies or hydrophobia. Now the true death-rate among persons thus bitten amounts to 15 per cent."—" *On Rabies*," *read before the Epidemiological Society, by Prof. V. Horsley*, Feb. 12th, 1889.

HYDROPHOBIA—Pasteur's Judgment on Nostrums for.

Pasteur.

LOUIS PASTEUR, Director of the Pasteur Institute, Paris. (V.)

"Now, suppose a hundred people to have been bitten by rabid dogs, how many will die of this terrible disease? It is difficult to answer such a question. Moreover, the number of victims varies for several reasons. Nevertheless, it is generally supposed that if the deaths taking place among a large number of persons bitten by rabid animals be added up, and if their seat and gravity be not taken into account, the mortality among persons bitten amounts to 15 or 20 per cent. In other words, more than 80 out of 100 persons suffer no evil effects from the bite. It is easy, therefore, to be deceived as to the value of any preventive remedy. For, if we apply it to a small number of persons, it will seem to have been successful in four cases out of five. Is that not more than sufficient to warrant a quack, whose advice is taken, to say that his remedy is infallible. and to cause ignorant men to blindly share his belief?"—*The New Review*, vol. i. p. 508 (Nov., 1889).

—— The same—Pasteur's a Quack· Remedy for.

Richards.

VINCENT RICHARDS (the late), F.R.C.S.Edin., M.R.C.S.Eng., Goalundo, Bengal. (V.)

" I have now advanced quite sufficient, and in language not too strong, to show that M. Pasteur's method of treatment, so far as the world has been enlightened, rests on no firmer basis than that which justified the vaunted powers of Holloway's Pills and Mother Seigel's Soothing Syrup."—*Hydrophobia and Pasteur* (Calcutta : Thacker and Spink, 1886), p. 20.

INFLAMMATION—The Phenomena of.

Macaulay.

JAMES MACAULAY, M.A., M.D., F.R.C.S.Ed., London. (A.V.)

" It is said in the *British Medical Journal* (p. 56, Jan. 9, 1875), 'Without vivisection-experiments we would know almost nothing of the phenomena of inflammation.' After all the observations of physicians and surgeons. of physiologists and pathologists, for successive generations, at home and abroad, we are told to look to vivisectors for almost all our knowledge of the causes, the symptoms, and the results of inflammation ! The plea is preposterous, and the fact of it being seriously put forward in an article specially written in defence of vivisection is sufficient to show the groundlessness of the alleged practical benefits of this method of research."—*Vivisection, A Prize Essay* (London, 1881), p. 50.

INOCULATIONS—Varying   "Medical Journal." Results of.

"THE BRITISH MEDICAL JOURNAL," Organ of the British Medical Association, London. (P.V.)

" M. Vulpian injected under the skin of rabbits saliva collected at the very moment of the experiment, from perfectly healthy individuals, and this injection killed the rabbit so inoculated in forty-eight hours. The blood of these rabbits was found to be filled with microscopic organisms ; among which was a special organism discovered by M. Pasteur in the course of his experiments with inoculation of the saliva of a child who had died of rabies. One drop of this blood, diluted in ten grammes of distilled water, and injected under the skin of other rabbits, also brought on the death of these animals, the blood of which was similarly filled with microscopic organisms. These singular results, of which the interpretation is by no means easy, present also the no less singular peculiarity of not being stable. Rabbits placed in identical conditions, and inoculated with the same saliva, experienced no ill effects from their inoculation, and continued in excellent health. It would therefore appear that experimental microbiology is not yet on the way to become either an easy or clear science, notwithstanding M. Pasteur's *fiat lux*."—*British Medical Journal*, April 9th, 1881, p. 571.

—— The same.—*See* SALIVA.

INSANITY—Failure of Vivisection to Relieve.   Gilbert.

WILLIAM GILBERT (the late), M.R.C.S., some time a Governor of Westminster Hospital (born 1804 ; died 1890). (A.V.)

" Among the most cruel of these experiments have been those on the brains of dogs and monkeys, not simply for surgical purposes, but, by far the most numerous, for cerebral diseases as well. And with what result ? The answer may be deduced from the following terrible facts. In the 13 general hospitals

L

in London, together with the principal special hospitals and the smallpox and fever hospitals, there are—medical and surgical cases combined—about 4,500 in-patients. In eight lunatic and idiot asylums there are no fewer than 13,420. Nor is this all. While there are many vacant beds in the hospitals, the lunatic and idiot asylums are not only full, but there are in the licensed houses and parish workhouses no fewer than 1,980 more waiting for admission, and these numbers are rapidly increasing. And yet of these patients, suffering from the most dreaded malady which can afflict humanity, and for whose benefit so many poor animals have died under vivisectional experiment, not in a single instance has it proved successful."— *Letter in " The Times,"* Dec. 30th, 1884.

INSPECTOR'S RETURNS—Value of the.   Harris.

STANFORD HARRIS, M.R.C.S., London. (A.V.)

"It may be worth while to give here a question of Mr. Forster's and the answer by Dr. Klein, as illustrating the foolishness of expecting men of the same profession to inspect one another (as is now the case under the Act). The humane minute issued from the Home Office was in this case rendered a dead letter.

"'Q. 3746. *Mr. Forster:* Do you recollect whether Mr. Simon informed you that when I was in office I had said something to them about this, or did he give you a minute that I wrote?—I think he spoke to me about it, but really it is so long ago that I could not be certain. Q. 3747: You cannot recollect whether he gave you a minute?—No. Q. 3748: You do not recollect his giving you any words written by me to this effect —" That no experiments on living animals should be conducted at the cost of the State without the employment of some anæsthetic in case of painful operations, and without a report from time to time by the gentleman conducting the experiments, explaining their object and showing the necessity for the purpose of discovery." Do you recollect seeing those words? —No. May I be allowed to say this, that at that time I was not connected directly with Mr. Simon. I was at that time simply an assistant of Dr. Burdon Sanderson, so that Mr. Simon could not have occasion to give me that instruction in an official way.' It further appears, however, that—(Q. 3749): 'When you were put directly under him, you had not that minute laid before you, as I understand you?—No.' "—*Darwin and the Royal Commission,* by S. Harris, M.R.C.S.

IPECACUANHA.　　　　　　　　　　　　Berdoe.

EDWARD BERDOE, M.R.C.S., L.R.C.P.Ed., London.　(A.V.)

"This is a favourite domestic remedy, and much used as an expectorant and emetic. Notwithstanding its enormous use, and the great number of experiments upon animals made with it by Orfila, Majendie, and later by Dr. Dyce Duckworth and others, 'its physiological action is not as yet well made out.'— (*Wood*, p. 431). The experiments of investigators indicate that the active principle of ipecacuanha (*emetia*) has very little action upon the lungs, but we know from daily observation that it is one of our most valuable and trustworthy expectorants.

"D'Ornellas and Pecholier are in opposition as to the action of *emetia* upon sensibility, the one affirming that it is not, the other that is, affected. They are not agreed as to its action on the temperature.—(*Wood*, p. 432)."—*The Futility of Experiments with Drugs on Animals*, by Edward Berdoe (London, 1889), pp. 25-6.

JABORANDI.　　　　　　　　　　　　　Berdoe.

EDWARD BERDOE, M.R.C.S, L.R.C.P.Ed., London.　(A.V.)

"Vulpian says that jaborandi does not slow the heart if curare be largely given so as to paralyse the vagus nerve. Mr. Langley (*Journal of Anatomy*, x. p. 188), showed the incorrectness of this by a series of similar experiments. Ever the same story!"—*The Futility of Experiments with Drugs on Animals*. by Edward Berdoe (London, 1889), p. 26.

KIDNEY REMOVAL, Operation for, not　　Berdoe.
due to Vivisection.

EDWARD BERDOE, M.R.C.S., L.R.C.P.Ed., London.　(A.V.)

"The operation for the removal of a diseased kidney was not discovered by experiments on animals. and even if it had been, there was no necessity for them, for the *post-mortem* table had proved that we can live with only one kidney. Let me refer your readers for proof of this to last week's *Lancet* (Dec., 1889), p. 1270, where Mr. Knowsley Thornton, in his lecture on the Surgery of the Kidneys, refers to 'the occasional absence of a second kidney, the knowledge that in one case at least (Polk's) a single kidney has been removed, the error only being discovered after the death of the patient.'"—*Letter in the* "*Bazaar*," Dec. 30th, 1889.

KIDNEY REMOVAL—Operation for, not   Macdonald.
due to Vivisection.

PETER WM. MACDONALD, M.D. and C.M., Aberd., Medical
Superintendent, Dorset County Asylum. (V.)

"Cases of congenital absence of one kidney are comparatively rare. Mr. Henry Morris, in an address before the
Medical Society of London, said: 'Out of 8068 *post-mortem*
cases there were but two instances of congenital absence, and
one only of congenital atrophy, of the kidney.' To have met
with two cases in less than one hundred necropsies has,
judging from recorded cases, been the experience of none."
[He then records details of two cases—one man and one
woman—where life had been sustained from birth with only
one kidney in each case ; thus showing that no vivisection
was necessary to prove that life can be maintained with but
one kidney to discharge the work of two in the functions of
the body.]—*The Lancet*, vol. i., 1885, pp. 979–80.

KNOWLEDGE OF SERVICE TO MAN—Is   Cobbe.
Vivisection capable of yielding?

FRANCES POWER COBBE, Authoress, Hengwrt, Dolgelly, N.
Wales. (A.V.)

"You ask first, Do we 'deny' that vivisection is capable of
yielding knowledge of service to man?' We are not so rash as
to deny that any practice, even the most immoral conceivable,
might possibly yield knowledge of service to man ; and, in
particular, we do not deny that the vivisection of human beings
by the surgeons of classic times, and again by the great anatomists of Italy in the 15th century, may very possibly have yielded
knowledge to man, and be capable, if revived, of yielding still
more.   We have, however, for a long time back called on the
advocates of the vivisection of dogs, monkeys, etc., to furnish
evidence of the beneficial results of their work, not as setting at
rest the question of its morality, but as an indispensable preliminary to justify them in coming into the court of public opinion
as defendants of a practice obviously (as the Royal Commissioners reported) 'liable from its very nature to great abuse,' and
involving transgression of the undoubted principles of English
law as embodied in the Act (12 and 13 Victoria, chap. 92) for the
general prevention of Cruelty to Animals.   At last, after the
lapse of several years, and after experiencing several 'false starts'
concerning tuberculosis, resection of the lungs, etc., we found a
few days ago, in your world-read columns, a formal answer to
our challenge. A gentleman, who did not give us his name, but
in a measure made himself the representative of science by

signing himself ' F.R.S.,' recounted a case which he described as ' unique,' wherein a patient's life had been preserved, and his wife and children saved from bereavement and penury by the aid of Professor Ferrier's experiments. We were preparing to argue the question of the morality of vivisection upon the basis of the ' unique ' case, when we received the intelligence that the poor patient's life was not saved after all, and that, as the *British Medical Journal* regretfully observes, ' F.R.S.'s' letter was an ' unfortunate indiscretion.' As we are too ' ignorant ' to take in all the scientific considerations whereby ' F.R.S.' in his second letter lets himself gently down from the altitude of the first, when he rebuked the Bishop of Oxford and Mr. Ruskin in a manner scarcely discreet, we must be excused if we now hold it to be demonstrated that whether vivisection be or be not ' capable of yielding useful knowledge,' it certainly yields only a scanty crop of it. Were there anything like an abundant harvest, such a sample as this would not have been produced with so much pomp for public scrutiny. In short, we think with Dr. Leffingwell that, ' if pain could be measured by money, there is no mining company in the world which would sanction prospecting in such barren regions.' "—*Letter in* " *The Times*," Dec. 30th, 1889.

KNOWLEDGE—How to obtain True. Fletcher.

JOHN FLETCHER, M.D., formerly Lecturer on Physiology and Medical Jurisprudence, Edinbro' Medical School. (A.V.)

" I am perfectly aware how much this plan of ' interrogating nature' has done, in modern times, for every branch of physical science: but I am equally persuaded that these advantages have been, in general, overrated—at any rate that students, in this respect generally begin at the wrong end, and are often engaged in experimenting on animals, in hope of finding out something or other on which to found some new and surprising doctrine, while they take no manner of notice of the great number of things continually going on in their own bodies, of the *rationale* of which they are ignorant. It was a precept which I learned from my first teacher in medicine, the late venerable Abernethy, constantly to remember that I carried always about with me the best subject for observation and experiment—one the most easily to be consulted, since it was quite in my power, and one the phenomena of which should be the most interesting to me, since it was with similar beings alone that I should in future have any immediate concern ; and this precept I have never lost sight of. We ought never to forget that the best subject for analysis is ourselves, and the most useful contemplation that which relates

to the most common processes; and that, till we understand all
which can be readily understood, with a little reflection, about
ourselves, and know the *rationalia* of all familiar phenomena,
it is preposterous to pore over the warm and quivering limbs of
other animals, in search of things recondite and comparatively
useless."—*Introductory Lecture (quoted in Dr. Macaulay's
Essay*, London, 1881, pp. 11, 12).

KNOWLEDGE, Not Utility, the Object of Vivisection. Hermann.

LUDIMAR HERMANN, Professor of Physiology and Medical
Physics, Zurich University. (V.)

" The advancement of our knowledge, and not utility to
medicine, is the true and straightforward object of all vivisection.
No true investigator in his researches thinks of the practical
utilization. Science can afford to despise this justification
with which vivisection has been defended in England."—*Die
Vivisectionsfrage für das grössere Publicum beleuchtet* (Leipsic,
1877).

—— Clinical and Pathological Study the True Source of.—
See CLINICAL AND PATHOLOGICAL STUDY.

—— Dearly bought by Vivisection. Johnson.

DR. SAMUEL JOHNSON, Author, etc. (born 1709; died 1784).
(A.V.)

" Among the inferior professors of medical knowledge is a
race of wretches whose lives are only varied by varieties of
cruelty; whose favourite amusement is to nail dogs to tables,
and then open them alive, to try how long life may be continued
in various degrees of mutilation or with the excision or laceration of the vital parts; to examine whether burning irons are
felt more acutely by bone or tendon; and whether the more
lasting agonies are produced by poisons forced into the mouth
or injected into the veins. It is not without reluctance that I
offend the sensibility of the tender mind with images like these.
If such cruelties were not practised, it were to be desired that
they should not be conceived, but since they are published
every day with ostentation, let me be allowed once to mention
them, since I mention them with abhorrence. . . . What is
alleged in defence of these hateful practices every one knows,
but the truth is that by knives, fire, and poisons, knowledge is
not always sought, and is very seldom attained. I know not
that by living dissections any discovery has been made by
which a single malady is more easily cured. And if the know-

.edge of physiology has been somewhat increased, he surely buys knowledge dear who learns the use of the lacteals at the expense of his own humanity. It is time that a universal resentment should arise against those horrid operations, which tend to harden the heart and make the physician more dreadful than the gout or the stone."—*The Idler*, No. 17.

KOCH—Scientific Opinion on his Treatment.   Williams.

C. THEODORE WILLIAMS, M.A., M.D., Consulting Physician to the Brompton Hospital. (V.)

" And now it will be seen that the evidence of the cases narrated does not confirm Professor Koch's conclusions, but like those of Prof. Virchow, Ewald, and Dr. C. J. Nixon, they point out some of the difficulties and dangers of the treatment. There is no doubt about the penetrative action of tuberculin, and possibly if something were combined with it this remarkable power of selecting tubercle might be turned to account ; as it stands at present in phthisis, its effect is to convert tuberculous masses, which may be perfectly quiescent, into cavities, and the process is by no means always a safe one. As regards the condition of our patients after treatment, all we can say is that they fared worse than the ordinary run of similar consumptives, and, moreover, that several of them improved considerably when transferred from Koch's system to the ordinary treatment of the hospital. There may be, and indeed there are, cases of phthisis in which the promotion of excavation is desirable, and for such the Koch method is indicated : but they are, I take it, exceedingly rare, and for the great mass of consumptive patients it is certainly not indicated."—" *The Treatment of Phthisis by Professor Koch's Method*." " *The Lancet* " (June 27th, 1891), p. 1417.*

—— The same—and Consumption.   Williams and Tatham.

CHARLES THEODORE WILLIAMS, M.D., F.R.C.P., Consulting Physician to the Consumption Hospital, Brompton ; and JOHN TATHAM, M.D. St. And., Consulting Physician to the Consumption Hospital, Brompton, London. (P.V.)

" The authorities of the Brompton Hospital for Consump-

* The *Family Doctor*, quoted in the *Court Circular*, Sept. 5, 1891, says: " The career of Koch's lymph as a specific for consumption has been brief." . . . Dr. L. S. Painter, of Pittsburg, Pa, expresses his opinion freely. " My experience was horrible. I am afraid they have killed me. They have killed them off in Berlin by hundreds. . . . Dr. Painter said that Prof. Virchow, who has performed hundreds of autopsies in lymph cures, has established the fact that instead of working as a cure the lymph will actually transfer tuberculosis throughout the whole system."

tion, desirous of doing everything that is humanly possible for the relief of the many sufferers from this direful disease, sanctioned their medical staff making a thorough practical experiment of the lymph in question [Koch's], feeling that if it possessed the merits ascribed to it by some, the results to mankind might be beneficial almost beyond belief. But un-fortunately the 'remedy' has now been proved to be as bad if not worse than the disease. Two of the most eminent specialists in chest diseases—Dr. Theodore Williams and Dr. Tatham—reporting as to the experiments, now state that the 'remedy' was used systematically for four months, during which time 30 patients were treated. After giving information as to the condition of the patients under treatment, the report concludes with these significant words :—'The tuberculin did not favourably influence the course of the disease in the majority of cases ; in some the effects were detrimental, and even in the stationary and improved cases it was difficult to ascribe any distinct improvement to the injections, which might not have been equally attained under the treatment ordinarily employed in the hospital.' We hope the public will now hesitate before giving credence to the dogmatic assertions of wonderful medical ' discoveries ' and ' cures ' by foreign doctors, and that at any rate the ghost has now been laid of the Koch ' cure ' which was heralded as little short of a miracle."—*The Globe* (London, January 13th, 1892).

LACTEALS, The.   Bell.

SIR   CHARLES   BELL,   M.R.C.S.   (the   late),   Lecturer   on
    Physiology, University College, London (born 1778 ; died
    1842). (V.)

" When the young anatomical student ties the mesenteric vessels of an animal recently killed, he finds the lacteals gradually swell ; he finds them turgid if the animal has had a full meal, and time has been afforded for the chyle to descend into the small intestines ; he finds them empty, or containing only a limpid fluid, if the animal has not had food. When he sees this he has had sufficient proof that these are the vessels for absorbing the nutritious fluids from the intestines. The actual demonstration of the absorbing mouths of the lacteal vessels is very difficult. The difficulty arises from these vessels being in general empty in the dead body, from the difficulty of injecting them from trunk to branch, in consequence of their valves ; and, lastly, from their orifices never being patent, except in a state of excitement. The anatomist must therefore watch

his opportunity when a man has been suddenly cut off in health, and after a full meal. Then the villi of the inner coat may be seen tinged with chyle, and their structure may be examined."
—*Lectures*, p. 360.

LACTEALS, The. Gimson.

GIMSON GIMSON, M.D. St. And., M.R.C.S., Witham, Essex. (A.V.)

" Lieberkühn and Cruikshank have been able to do this ; the latter opened a woman who had died suddenly of convulsions after taking a hearty supper in perfect health. 'Many of the villi,' he says, 'were so full of chyle that I saw nothing of the ramifications of the arteries and veins ; the whole appeared as one white vesicle, without any red lines, pores, or orifices what-ever. Others of the villi contained chyle, but in a small pro-portion, and the ramifications of the veins were numerous, and prevailed by their redness over the whiteness of the villi.'" (Elliotson, p. 123.)—*Vivisections and Painful Experiments on Living Animals, etc.* (London, 1879), p. 124.

LEAD. Berdoe.

EDWARD BERDOE, M.R.C.S., L.R.C.P.Ed., London. (A.V.)

" ' The muscular action of lead in poisonous doses is exceed-ingly pronounced in rabbits, but is feeble in dogs and cats.'—(*Wood*, p. 38.)

" Lead poisoning in man often produces loss of sensation and obscurity of vision, but Stillé says (p. 1,116), 'Experiments upon animals throw no light upon the occurrence of anæs-thesia, amaurosis, etc., from lead.'"—*The Futility of Experi-ments with Drugs on Animals*, by Edward Berdoe (London, 1889), p. 36.

LIFE, SAVING AND PROLONGATION OF, Macaulay.
· due to Causes other than Vivisection.

JAMES MACAULAY, M.A., M.D., F.R.C.S.Ed., London. (A.V.)

" After the middle of last century the mortality of children under five years of age, in London, was about fifty in the hundred. It is now not more than from thirty to thirty-five. The saving of life by improvement in the hygiene and manage-ment of infancy is now more than 100,000 human beings a year throughout Great Britain. The average mortality at all ages, and especially in towns, has remarkably decreased ; and the chances of life have steadily increased. Some of the diseases which were formerly among the most fatal in the bills of mortality, scurvy, dysentery, ague, and smallpox, are now low in the lists. The treatment of actual disease is only one department of practical medicine. The preservation of health and the prolongation of life are equally important. These objects are attained on the large scale by the prevention of disease much more than by its cure."—*Vivisection, A Prize Essay* (London, 1881), p. 20.

LIGATURE OF ARTERIES.   Macaulay.

JAMES MACAULAY, M.A., M.D., F.R.C.S.Ed., London.   (A.V.)

" The improvement in the mode of the ligature of arteries, introduced early in this century by Mr. Jones, has been ascribed to experiments on animals. These experiments may have confirmed his views, and satisfied others who saw them, but they were made in support of observation in the human body, which a few trials on small vessels, in the operating theatre, would have established far more speedily and surely. Yet this was presented by one witness to the Royal Commission as proving the necessity for experiments."—*Vivisection, A Prize Essay* (London, 1881), p. 68.

LISTERISM.—*See* Antiseptic Surgery.

LIVER—The Glycogenic Function of the.   Macaulay.

JAMES MACAULAY, M.A., M.D., F.R.C.S.Ed., London.   (A.V.)

" The glycogenic function of the liver has been much vaunted as an important contribution to physiological knowledge, applicable to improvement in medical practice. Mr. Erichsen, as spokesman of the Commissioners, made the most of it in taking the evidence of Professor Turner. ' In diabetes it was supposed, not many years ago, that the sugar was formed in the kidneys ; it is now known by physiological experiment that the sugar may be produced by a lesion of the nervous system. Claude Bernard has shown that, if a certain portion of the brain is injured, you get sugar in the urine ; that the sugar has nothing more to do with the kidney, and is no more a kidney disease, in point of fact, than the purulent expectoration in a consumptive patient has to do with the mouth ; that the kidney merely evolves it from the system, just as the mouth ejects the purulent matter from the lungs ? ' To which Professor Turner replied, ' That is the case ' (3,126). Mr. Erichsen's question was evidently framed for the instruction of his non-

professional colleagues of the Commission.   The analogy sug·
gested between the expulsion of diabetic sugar by the kidney
and of purulent sputa by the mouth was rather a strong figure
of speech; but, passing this, it was scarcely right of Mr.
Erichsen and Mr. Turner to make the Commissioners suppose
that ' not many years ago sugar was believed to be formed in
the kidneys.'   As long ago as the time of Dr. Mead, that distinguished physician ascribed the diabetic urine to a morbid
state of the liver and bile. A century ago Dr. Cullen taught that
the morbid state of the urine arose from the disorder of the
nutritive and assimilative functions connected with the diges·
tive system.   This was received by the profession generally;
and the melituria was understood to indicate an abnormal
result of animal chemistry, one process of which, in natural
health, was the production of sugar.   What Bernard showed
was, that the formation of sugar in the liver in the normal
state is so constant that the liver may be regarded as the
sugar-producing organ.   He demonstrated this by numerous
observations, especially by examining the livers of seven
recently-dead human subjects.   Five of these were executed
criminals.

*   *   *   *   *

   " All the experiments go no further than to show that the
normal secretion of sugar depends on healthy action of the
organs engaged in nutrition ; while unnatural interference with
the actions of these organs, especially by lesion of the nervous
centres by which their action is sustained, produces abnormal
secretion of sugar, and diabetes.   This multitude of experiments I regard as unjustifiable and needless cruelties, and
leading to no useful result."—*Vivisection, A Prize Essay* (London, 1881), pp. 44-5.

LUNG—Resection of.—*See* RESECTION OF LUNG.

MEDICAL PROFESSION, THE, Not   Macaulay.
well up on Vivisection.

JAMES MACAULAY, M.A., M.D., F.R.C.S.Ed., London.   (A.V.)

   " I put the question lately to the senior physician of one of
our great London hospitals, if he thought vivisection had
added anything to our resources which might not have been
otherwise obtained, and his reply was that he had not studied
the matter so as to give an answer.   Another physician,
occupying one of the highest positions in the profession, on
my asking him about some alleged physiological discoveries,

said he must inquire from his friend, P. S——, naming a surgeon and experimenter of Guy's Hospital. In the same way I have tested other medical friends, and find they are at a loss to name any practical benefits derived from vivisection. They are told that important investigations are instituted, and they are unwilling to object to any mode of research which is said to give promise of results. Comparatively few have personally studied the question, or have ventured openly to express doubt or disapproval."—*Vivisection, A Prize Essay* (London, 1881), p. 19.

MEDICAL PROFESSION, THE, Not well up on Vivisection. Arnold.

F. S. ARNOLD, M.B., B.Ch. (Oxon), M.R.C.S., Manchester. (A.V.)

" The great bulk of medical opinion on the subject of experiments on animals, on the other hand, is a largely uninstructed opinion. The question whether medicine and surgery have or have not benefited by vivisection, is one that requires separate study, and not one in one hundred of those medical men who give mechanical votes in favour of vivisection at meetings of the British Medical Association and elsewhere, and think no terms of abuse too offensive to hurl at the heads of anti-vivisectionists, has given the slightest special attention, or can engage in arguments on the utilitarian, to say nothing of the moral aspect of the question, without making the most absurd and preposterous blunders."—*From a Paper read at the Church Congress*, 1892.

—— The same. Benefits to, claimed for Vivisection. Macaulay.

JAMES MACAULAY, M.A., M.D., F.R.C.S.Ed., London. (A.V.)

" In an article in the *British Medical Journal* (January, 1875), entitled ' What has Vivisection done for Humanity ? ' the following are the examples given, under the head of benefits, in ' advancing therapeutics, relief of pain,' etc. :—1. Use of ether. 2. Use of chloroform. 3. Chloral discovered experimentally by Liebreich. 4. The action of all remedies are only definitely ascertained by experiments on animals. 5. Action of Calabar Bean by Fraser. 6. Antagonism between active substances and the study of antidotes.—Many observers.

" Could there be a more meagre and more misleading set of examples ? The practical use of anæsthetics would have been introduced and perfected if a single experiment on an inferior animal had never been made. The action of remedies on the human body can only be definitely ascertained by observation, and experiments on animals are more likely to mislead than to assist in gaining this definite knowledge. The action of some substances, such as antimony on horses and mercury on dogs. is widely different from their action on the human subject ; and the effects, both of remedies and of poisons, vary much in the different animals experimented on. Dr. Thorowgood says he has seen opium given to a pigeon, enough to kill a strong man. without any effect. Goats have been known to browse on tobacco leaves, and rabbits on belladonna, without harm. Many such anomalies have been observed, and the only certain knowledge of the influence of substances on the human subject must be obtained by observation of cases in private or in hospital practice."—*Vivisection, A Prize Essay* (London, 1881), pp. 48-9.

MEDICINE, Physicians' Testimony against the Benefit of Vivisection in. Macaulay.

JAMES MACAULAY, M.A., M.D., F.R.C.S.Ed., London. (A.V.)

" If the testimony of physicians of the highest rank in the profession is accepted, their verdict is against the alleged benefits of vivisection in the practice of the healing art. Sir James Y. Simpson did not even allude to it, in enumerating the causes of the advancement of medicine and surgery during the last half-century. Professor Newman says : ' I can attest that Dr. James Cowles Prichard assured me that vivisection had added nothing whatever to the physician's power of healing.' When Sir Thomas Watson was giving evidence before the Royal Commission, the question was asked : ' Although you have never performed any experiments, nor witnessed them, you have used the results of the experiments of others. have you not, as the basis for the advancement of your professional knowledge?' The answer was : ' I have made myself acquainted with the experiments and their results, and have turned them to such uses as I could.' Of this reply Mr. Macilwain. himself a distinguished and experienced surgeon, in reviewing the evidence, says : ' Could any answer convey a more measured recognition of a mode of study, in reply to the question whether he had not made it a *basis* for the advancement of his professional knowledge ? Could anything be more vague or unsatisfactory ? Why was so experienced a witness not requested to favour the Commission with some of the details of so vast an experience ? Why was he not requested to state in *what* cases he had turned it to account, and how far it had or had not answered his expectations ? ' The truth is, that the question was put apparently for the sake of the lay members of the Commission, and for the non-professional readers of the Blue Book. It was intended to suggest that vivisection had been the source of improvements, if not of an entire reform of practice, in thus speaking of it as *the basis of advance in professional knowledge.* The interrogator knew too well, however, how imprudent it would be to follow up the tentative question. To have asked for details or examples would have exposed the futility of the claims of the vivisectionists to have amended or altered medical practice. Where attempts have been made to give details, the examples are not only few, but they lead at once back to the very matter under dispute, whether the knowledge on which the practice rests came from vivisection or from legitimate methods of research."—*Vivisection, A Prize Essay* (London, 1881), pp. 47-8.

MERCURIAL SALTS (as Calomel,   Berdoe. Bichloride of Mercury, etc.).

EDWARD BERDOE, M.R.C.S., L.R.C.P.Ed., London. (A.V.)

"' The experience of generations strongly supports,' says Dr. Ringer (*Materia Medica*, 12th Ed., p. 243), ' the general conviction that in some diseases calomel, as well as other preparations of mercury, does increase the bile.' But Drs. Hughes-Bennett and Rutherford performed a very large number of cruel and excessively painful experiments on the livers of dogs. The abdomen was cut open, and a glass tube tied into the bile duct, with barbarous attendant circumstances, which placed the animals in an abnormal condition ; mercurials and other drugs were inserted in the cut intestines to show their effects. The operators came to the conclusion that the doctors had been all wrong in their conclusions about calomel, and they proved to their own satisfaction that it did not increase the secretion of the bile. Of course no physician worthy of the name paid the slightest attention to these conclusions, but went on administering what his experience had proved to be so valuable ; and fortunately so, for it ultimately dawned upon the intellects of Messrs. Bennett and Rutherford that there was all the difference between administering calomel by the stomach—thereby mixing it with the gastric juice—and cutting open the upper part of the intestines and inserting the drug there. Rutherford also found that the curare given to keep the animals quiet, diminished the bile and made the heart's action weak and irregular."—*The Futility of Experiments with Drugs on Animals*, by Edward Berdoe (London, 1889), p. 27.

MERCY TO ANIMALS—A Christian Virtue.
Chalmers.

THE REV. DR. CHALMERS (born 1780 ; died 1847). (A.V.)

" Humanity is a virtue which oversteps, as it were, the limits of a species, and which prompts a descending movement on our part, of righteousness and mercy towards those who have an inferior place to ourselves in the scale of creation. It is not the circulation of benevolence within the limits of one species. It is the transmission of it from one species to another. The first is but the charity of a world. The second is the charity of a universe. Had there been no such charity, no descending current of love and of compassion from species to species, what, I ask, should have become of ourselves ? . . . The distance upward between us and that mysterious Being who let Himself down from Heaven's high concave upon our lowly platform, surpasses by infinity the distance downward between us and everything that breathes. And he bowed Himself thus far for the purpose of an example, as well as for the purpose of an expiation, that every Christian might extend his compassionate regards over the whole of sentient and suffering nature."—*From " Cruelty to Animals,"* a Sermon preached in Edinburgh by the Rev. T. Chalmers, D.D. (March 5, 1826).

MISLEADING—Vivisection has done more to perpetuate Error than to confirm Just Views.
Bell.

SIR CHARLES BELL (the late), M.R.C.S. London, Sen. Prof. Anat. Surg. Roy. Coll. Surg. Lond., and M.C., 1824 ; Lect. Physiol. Univ. Coll. Lond., 1826 ; knighted 1831 ; Prof. Surg. Univ. Edin., 1831 (born 1778 ; died 1842). (V.)

" In concluding these papers, I hope I may be permitted to offer a few words in favour of anatomy, as better adapted for discovery than experiment. Anatomy is already looked upon with prejudice by the thoughtless and ignorant ; let not its professors unnecessarily incur the censures of the humane. Experiments have never been the means of discovery ; and a survey of what has been attempted of late years in physiology, will prove that the opening of living animals has been done more to perpetuate error than to confirm the just views taken from the study of anatomy and natural motions. In a foreign

review of my former papers the results have been considered
as a further proof in favour of experiments. They are, on the
contrary, deductions from anatomy, and I have had recourse
to experiments, not to form my own opinions, but to impress
them upon others. It must be my apology that my utmost
efforts of persuasion were lost while I urged my statements on
the grounds of anatomy alone."—*Nervous System of the Human
Body* (Longmans & Co., 1839), p. 217.

MISLEADING.   Ferrier.

DAVID FERRIER, M.D.Edin., 1870 ; F.R.C.P.Lond., 1877 ;
    M.D., 1872 ; F.R.S., Professor of Neuropathy, King's College,
    London.   (V.)

" Experiments on the lower animals, even on apes, often
lead to conclusions seriously at variance with well-established
facts of clinical and pathological observation. . . . The
decisive settlement of such points must depend mainly on
careful clinical and pathological research. . . . Experiments have led to different views in different hands."
—Ferrier's " *Functions of the Brain* " (Preface).

—— The same—and Degrading.   Gooding.

JAS. C. GOODING, M.D.Ed., M.R.C.S.Eng., Cheltenham.   (A.V.)

" I have never myself, either when a student in London or
Edinburgh, seen a vivisection experiment ; and believe that
they turn into a wrong channel observation and inferences
which would find more fruitful and less bewildering results in
other directions.   Did history not give us plenty of record, one
would wonder how the human mind could descend to such
depths of degradation as is evidenced by some of the experiments recorded by vivisectionists."—*Letter to Miss Hanson*,
Dec. 31st, 1884.

—— The same.   Longet.

FRANÇOIS ACHILLE LONGET, late Professor of Physiology at
    the Medical Faculty of Paris.   (V.)

" Experiments on animals of a different species, so far from
leading to useful results as regarded human beings, had a
tendency to mislead us.   In seeking to benefit mankind by
vivisections, it would be necessary to have recourse to
pathological facts founded on experiments on *human* beings."
—*Longet, quoted in Fleming's Essay*, p. 42.

MISLEADING.   Macilwain.

GEORGE MACILWAIN (the late), F.R.C.S., a Witness before the
Royal Commission, 1875 (born 1827 ; died 1882). (A.V.)

"We understand you to say that you mention the case
of Mr. Travers's experiments upon animals in regard to
strangulated hernia as a proof that such experiments may
not only not lead in the right direction. but may be absolutely
misleading ?—Yes ; if you add to that, and the practice he
deduced from them.

  * * * * *

"You practised vivisection many years ago yourself, I
understand you to say ?—I did a little. but that was very early
indeed.
"Your view is that vivisection is wholly useless, and worse
than useless ?—It is."—*Evid. Royal Com.* (London, 1876),
Q. 1,852-54.

—— The same.   Macilwain.

GEORGE MACILWAIN, F.R.C.S. (the late), a witness before the
Royal Commission, 1875 (born 1797 ; died 1882). (A.V.)

"So far has vivisection been from helping us at the bedside
of the patient—it is a fact. beyond all controversy. that it has
led to most serious errors ; nay, sometimes to inferences which,
were the subject not too grave, would be held as absurd and
ridiculous."—*Remarks, Logical and Physiological, on Vivisection*, 1860.

—— The same.   Tait

LAWSON TAIT, F.R.C.S., late Professor of Gynæcology, Queen's
College, Birmingham. (A.V.)

"Simpson, in the year 1862 I think it was, set me to work
under his direction to discover a better means than we had of
arresting the hæmorrhage in these cases, and as was the
fashion of those days, and is too much the fashion of these
days now, we turned our attention first and foremost to experiments upon the lower animals, and in one of the medical
journals. the *Medical Times and Gazette* for the year 1863 or
1864. there is described in detail a long series of experiments
which I performed under Simpson's directions upon all sorts
of animals, in order to secure this result. The results were
extremely satisfactory ; that is to say, by an ingenious contrivance which Simpson brought into use, I got conclusions

which were in themselves quite satisfactory. Thus in an experiment upon a dog, it was very easy to get the bleeding to stop ; sometimes, in fact, we could not get the arteries to bleed at all in the dog ; but when we came to the treatment of human beings, it was a different thing altogether. The artery would not stop bleeding by our means, and the conclusion of our experiments upon animals was that they could not be applied to human beings, and the whole thing was a failure. Those experiments, as far as I am personally concerned—and the author of the paper I am now discussing will admit that with my name goes a great deal of the history of the matter— those experiments kept us back twelve years."—*Speech at the Annual Meeting, London Society, St. James's Hall, May 26th*, 1891.

MISLEADING.   Jones.

T. WHARTON JONES (the late), F.R.C.S., F.R.S., formerly Prof. of Ophthalmological Med. and Surg. Univ. Coll. Hospital (born 1808 ; died 1891). (V.)

"The experiments on living animals which have been performed in order to prove the existence of vaso-dilator nerves and a mechanism on which they exert their excito-motor influence are utterly inconclusive, little better than gambling in vivisection with the expectation of eliciting something by chance, and betray on the part of the experimenters a want of fundamental acquaintance with the mechanism of the circulation in the extreme vessels, and with the different parts played therein by the small arteries, capillaries, and venous radicles. Thus it is that experiments are sometimes performed on living animals in order to ascertain the special action of nerves without a preliminary acquaintance with the mechanism of the organ, the nervous influence on which constitutes the subject of research ; nay, experiments are performed in order to demonstrate the action of supposed nerves of imaginary organs, of which the existence is assumed in order to account for inaccurately observed phenomena. And all this is dignified by the name of 'experimental research,' while such crucial facts as the directly observable mechanism by which the flow of blood is promoted in the veins of the bats' wing, and the remarkable phenomenon attending the propulsion of lymph from the lymphatic heart in the eel's tail into the caudal vein are unstudied and stupidly misrepresented."—"*Dilatation of the Calibre of Small Arteries,*" *Lancet*, November 15th, 1884 (pp. 864-7).

—— **The Same.**—*See* SUPPOSITION—MACAULAY.

MORAL ASPECTS—Animals "must suffer to save man's pain." Cobbe.

FRANCES POWER COBBE, Authoress, Hengwrt, Dolgelly, North Wales. (A.V.)

" To affirm, then, as vivisectors are wont to do, that they would freely ' sacrifice a hecatomb of dogs to save the smallest pain of a man,' is merely an expression of contempt for the rights of beings feebler than themselves, and which are not yet advanced by evolution to the lordly class of ' Bimana,' or the genus ' Homo.' What are the moral grounds, we ask, for this astounding new principle of *Race Selfishness* ? What is there in man, either considered only as our fellow-bimanous animal, or as an immortal being whose body is but the garment of his soul, which should make his trifling pain so inexpressibly solemn a matter, and the agony of another animal, no less physically sensitive, insignificant by comparison ? Of course we may naturally feel a little more spontaneous sympathy with a suffering man than with a suffering horse. But what is the ethical reason why we should prefer the pain of a thousand horses to that of a single man ? Sir Henry Taylor has written noble lines on this matter, going deep into the heart of the question :—

> ' Pain, terror, mortal agonies that scare
> Thy heart in man, to brutes thou wilt not spare :
> Are theirs less sad and real ? *Pain in man*
> *Bears the high mission of the flail and fan ;*
> *In brutes 'tis purely piteous.*'*

" There is no sight in all the world, to a thoughtful mind, more suggestive of harrowing reflection, no line of the long ' riddle of the painful earth ' more confounding to the religious soul, than the sufferings of creatures who have never sinned, and for whom (according to common belief) there will be no compensation for injustice in another life. While human pain has its plausible explanations and its possible beneficent results, animal pain seems (at least to our dim eyes) sheer unmitigated evil. I am at a loss then to conceive on what principle, deserving the name of moral, we are to speak and act as if such evil counted absolutely for nothing, while the aches and pains of men are to be so highly esteemed, that the most cruel sacrifices must not be spared, if a chance exist of alleviating them. When we remember who are the teachers who talk about the ' hecatomb,' and what is their view of the

* Poems: Vol. III. "The Amphitheatre at Pozzuoli."

relationship of man to the lower animals, we discover (as above remarked) that the only intelligible principle on which they proceed is that very ancient one—*le droit du plus fort*. As the main work of civilization has been the vindication of the rights of the weak, it is not too much, I think, to insist that the practice of vivisection, in which this tyranny of strength culminates, is a retrograde step in the progress of our race ; a backwater in the onward flowing stream of justice and mercy, no less portentous than deplorable."—*The Moral Aspects of Vivisection*, 6th ed. (London, 1884), pp. 17, 18.

MORAL ASPECTS, THE—The End does not   Clark. necessarily justify the Means.

THOMAS BEAVAN CLARK, Edgbaston, Birmingham.   (A.V.)

" Mr. G. J. Romanes, in the *Times* of the 20th January, writes :—' In cases where there is presumably a large disproportion between the necessary suffering entailed by the means and the prospective benefit to be secured by the end, the means are morally justified, even when the suffering is inflicted upon man—a truth which is recognised alike in surgery. in criminal law, and even in the punishment of children.'

    *   *   *   *   *

"As a matter of fact, is this 'truth' thus 'recognised ?'   In surgery do we sacrifice one man's leg, in order that another man's life may be saved ?   In criminal law do we put one innocent man in prison in order that twenty other men may be deterred from crime ?   Do we punish an innocent child in order that his naughty brothers and sisters may be conscience-stricken ?   Of course we do not.

    *   *   *   *   *

" We all recognise that it is moral for a man to sacrifice his own leg to save his own life, for the life is more to him than the leg ; ' there is, presumably, a large disproportion between the suffering and the prospect of benefit to be secured ; ' but, then, by a curious feat of argumentative legerdemain, Mr. Romanes proceeds to argue that you may, with equal morality, cut off the man's leg to save another man's life, or torture a score of dogs to save a hundred lives, because still, 'there is, presumably, a large disproportion between the suffering and the prospect of benefit to be secured.'   And I find that many simple-minded readers conclude that that also must be right, not in the least perceiving that the conjuror has changed the balls.   If it be unjust to forcibly sacrifice one man's life, in order to save one other man's life (which I suppose even Mr. Romanes would admit), then it must still be unjust to do so in order to save the lives of two, ten, or twenty others—that is, unjust to the man sacrificed. So we contend injustice to an animal is not lessened by the fact of any number of other animals, human or otherwise, benefiting by the injustice."— *Letter in " The Times,"* Jan. 22nd, 1885.

MORAL ASPECTS—The Rudiments of Virtue.   Cobbe.

FRANCES POWER COBBE, Authoress, Hengwrt, Dolgelly, North Wales. (A.V.)

" Are we not altogether on a wrong track in arguing this question on the level to which we have descended ? Are not generosity, self-sacrifice, the readiness to suffer, the very rudiments of all virtue and all nobility of character ? Are we to go back to the condition of savages—nay, rather of those

> ' Dragons of the prime
> Which tare each other in their slime,'

when we have boasted we had ascended to the rank of men, of Christians. of English gentlemen ? Is it a question for a man who aspires to be a brave or worthy, not to speak of a chivalrous or noble person, whether he *may*, within the limits of actual offence, spend his days in putting harmless animals on the rack for the benefit of himself and his kind ? And is it our proper teachers, those who are fit to guide and train young minds, and direct the tendencies of future generations, who are striving to move us to condone and approve such deeds by cant about the ' Glory of Science,' and by appeals to our miserable, cowardly fears of disease, and our selfish willingness to save 'the smallest pain of a man at the cost of the torture of a hecatomb of brutes ' ? To me it appears, I avow, that all this reveals a backsliding in feeling and moral aim almost measureless in the depth of its descent. The whole notion of vivisection, as a legitimate exercise and mode of satisfying human desire of knowledge, seems to rest on a radically false conception of the proper ends of human life, and a no less erroneous idea of our relationship to those humbler tribes of creatures who are our fellow-lodgers in this planet-house of the Almighty. As life is more than meat, so are there better things to live for than knowledge or escape from pain ; nor is any fact which science can reveal worth acquiring at the price of selfishness and cruelty."—*The Moral Aspects of Vivisection,* 6th ed. (London, 1884), p. 19.

MORAL ASPECTS—Man's Duty to the Brutes.   Cobbe.

FRANCES POWER COBBE, Authoress, Hengwrt, Dolgelly, North Wales. (A.V.)

" If we deal first with the ethical side of that question, do we not find something very like the following syllogism ?

" 1. Man owes *some* duty to the brutes as sentient beings ; and the *minimum* at which such duty can be assessed is to refrain from inflicting on them the *very worst* they can be made to suffer.

" 2. Vivisection frequently involves the infliction on brutes of the very worst they can suffer.

" 3. Therefore, such (worst) vivisection is a dereliction from man's duty to the brutes, as sentient creatures.

" I confess I do not see how this conclusion is to be evaded save by denying the major proposition, and affirming that man owes duty only to his equals in the scale of existence— a doctrine equivalent to saying that a gentleman need only behave as such to other gentlemen, but with his inferiors may blamelessly be a bully and a cad."—*Letter in " The Speaker "* (London, July, 1891).

—— The same—Impossible to separate Lawful from Unlawful Vivisection.   Freeman.

EDWARD A. FREEMAN, M.A. (the late), Regius Professor of Modern History, University of Oxford (died 1892). (A.V.)

"I presume that physiologists themselves would find it hard to draw the line between experiments done directly to relieve suffering and experiments done in the ordinary pursuit of know-ledge. It would certainly be hard to draw the same kind of line in any other branch of study.

         *   *   *

" The practical conclusion that I come to is that if the distinc-tion can be drawn in practice between what I hold to be lawful and unlawful vivisection, I would allow one and forbid the other. But I see the very great difficulty in drawing the line between the two ; and, if it cannot be drawn in practice, especially as it seems so very doubtful whether vivisection has lessened human suffering or not, I can only go in for a complete forbidding of the practice."—*Letter in " The Times,"* Jan. 16th, 1885.

MORAL ASPECTS—Compassion lost in   Mackarness. the Vivisector.

BISHOP MACKARNESS (the late), of Oxford (born 1820; died 1889). (A.V.)

" I am quite sure I am justified in saying this, because it is a matter of wide experience, that one strong emotion in the human mind will so absorb as to exclude another,—nay, even all other emotions,—so long as it lasts. The miser has lost the perception of suffering, which he might relieve, in his absolute devotion to the accumulation of gold. The sensualist may lose the power of appreciating the misery and shame his profligacy causes ; and so with the physiologist. He is so absorbed in the work, and his desire for knowledge, that he is incapable of appreciating the pain which he causes ; he has, in point of fact, put that matter entirely out of court. I do not say that when he is carrying on his work he desires to give unnecessary pain, but he is so absorbed that he does not know the nature or the extent of the torture he inflicts. Now see then what the result is—what the terrible result is we are brought to by this devotion to the higher duty, as Dr. Playfair describes it. We are brought really to this result, that we get rid of the feeling of compassion from men's nature and lose the influence and power of it. Yet this power is one of the greatest safeguards to weakness, and the protection against unnumbered crimes of violence. The would-be perpetrator of a crime is often moved at the last moment by that feeling of compassion which he thought he had got rid of, but which rises within him and stays his hand. To get rid of compassion is to get rid of one of the most lovely and refining virtues of the human character. God forbid that we should attempt to abolish one of His noblest gifts."—*Speech at Annual Meeting of the Victoria Street and International Society* (London, May 1st, 1883), p. 6.

—— The same—Duty to Man before   Mackarness. Duty to Beasts.

BISHOP MACKARNESS (the late), of Oxford (born 1820; died 1889). (A.V.)

" The assertion of Dr Lyon Playfair, which is quoted in the 15th page of the ' Comments on the Debate,' is this—' Man's duty to man is greater than his duty to beasts,' and upon that is founded a very serious argument in favour of vivisection. Now I suppose the assertion, if it be rightly understood, is one which no one would dispute, but then I am bound to add that

it is one which is not very likely to be understood rightly, and I could go further and say that it is more likely than not to be misunderstood. Let us for a moment vary the statement and take a different class of duty altogether. Suppose we say that the duty of any one to his parent is higher than his duty to a stranger—that is indisputable. Filial duty is that which regulates our conduct in the earliest part of our lives, and it is imprinted in our nature; if we disregarded that duty, home and family ties would be destroyed. But it does not follow that our duties towards a stranger are therefore abolished. There may be cases in which a man's duty to a stranger may even prevail over his duty to his parent. I may be required to give some assistance to a needy parent, but would justice say that I should do so if I owed the money as a debt to a stranger? I must pay my debt to that stranger as duty calls upon me to do. That is obvious; and in fact the further you go into Dr. Lyon Playfair's statement, as I have read it, it will appear that the duties which he compares together do not afford materials for comparison. If I suppose the case of a human being suffering from some temporary ailment or pain, and an animal dying from thirst. it would be my duty to give a cup of water to the dying creature before I attended to the trifling ailment of the man. What we have to do is to consider the urgency and the need of the case, as well as the quality of the object."
—*Speech at Annual Meeting of the Victoria Street and International Society*, May 1st (London, 1883), pp. 3, 4.

MORAL ASPECTS—Duty to Man before Duty to Beasts.   ·   Cobbe.

FRANCES POWER COBBE, Authoress, Hengwrt, Dolgelly.   (A.V.)

" Dr. Playfair makes a great display of ethical philosophy in laying down the canon,

' Man's duty to man is greater than his duty to beasts.'

" I entirely concur in the principle, but I consider that it requires those who hold it to prohibit vivisection. Man's paramount duty to man is founded on the fact of the moral nature of man, and, consequently, regards, primarily and before all others, the interests of that moral nature. We are required by the highest ethics to seek the moral benefit of our brother before his physical welfare; his *Virtue* before his *Happiness*. This being the case, we must endeavour to stop a practice injurious to the moral interests of humanity. Vivisection is unquestionably thus injurious to the moral interests of humanity, irrespective of the contention whether it be, or be not, conducive to any physical advantage."—*Comments on the Debate in the House of Commons*, April 4th, 1883, by Frances Power Cobbe (London, 1883), p. 15.

MORAL ASPECTS—The True Sense of   Ruskin.   Feeling.

JOHN RUSKIN, (then) Slade Professor of Fine Art, Oxford University. (A.V.)

" It was not the question whether experiments taught them more or less of science. It was not the question whether animals had a right to this or that in the inferiority they were placed in to mankind. It was a question—What relation had they to God, what relation mankind had to God, and what was the true sense of feeling as taught to them by Christ the Physician? The primary head and front of all the offending against both the principle of mercy in men and the will of the Creator of these creatures was the ignoring of that will in higher matters, and these scientific pursuits were now defiantly, provokingly, insultingly separated from the science of religion ; they were all carried on in defiance of what had hitherto been held to be compassion and pity, and of the great link which bound together the whole of creation from its Maker to the lowest creature. For one secret discovered by the torture of a thousand animals, a thousand means of health, peace, and happiness were lost, because the physician was continually infecting his students, not with the common rabies of the dog, but with the rabies of the man, infecting them with all kinds of base curiosity, infecting the whole society which he taught with a thirst for knowing things which God had concealed from them for His own good reason, and promoting amongst them passions of the same kind."—*Speech at Oxford*, December 9th, 1884.

—— The same—Revelation and   Shaftesbury.   Vivisection.

THE EARL OF SHAFTESBURY, K.G. (the late), (born 1801 ; died 1885). (A.V.)

" Whether the law was efficient or inefficient, whether vivisection was conducive to science or the reverse, there was one great preliminary consideration : On what authority of Scripture, or any other form of revelation, he asked most solemnly, did they rest their right to subject God's creatures to such unspeakable sufferings ? The thought had troubled the mind of many vivisectors ; it had deeply touched the heart of Sir Charles Bell. That they might take the life of animals for food, or to remove danger or annoyance, he fully admitted; but he utterly denied that they were permitted to indulge their curiosity or even advance their knowledge by the infliction of exquisite torture on the sentient creation. They were told in haughty and dogmatic style that the secrets of nature could be learnt in no other way. Learned in no other way ! Could it be believed that the Almighty had issued such a decree ? The animals were His creatures as much as we were His creatures ; and 'His tender mercies,' so the Bible told us, 'were over all His works.' He, along with many, repudiated such an atrocious and shallow doctrine ; and under that conviction he would ever do his best to put down a system that was as needless as it was cruel."—*Speech in support of Lord Truro's Bill, House of Lords*, 15th July, 1879.

MORALITY, Science must not disregard.   Stephen

LESLIE STEPHEN, Esq., Author, London.   (R.)

" We are bound to see that the sacred name of science is not used as a shelter for unworthy practices. When the country is asked to become more scientific, it must be shown that the demand does not involve the very slightest disregard for the common principles of morality. True knowledge and morality must progress together if, as scientific men tell us, morality must be based upon a thorough understanding of the conditions of human welfare."—*From " The Ethics of Vivisection," " Cornhill Magazine,"* April, 1876.

MORAL TRUST, Man's Dominion over   Erskine.
Animals a.

LORD ERSKINE (the late), Lord Chancellor of England, 1806 (born 1750 ; died 1823). (A.V.)

" That the dominion of man over the lower world is a moral trust, is a proposition which no man living can deny, without denying the whole foundation of our duties. If, in the examination of these qualities, powers, and instincts of animals, we could discover nothing else but their admirable and wonderful construction for man's assistance ; if we found no organs in the animals for their own gratification and happiness—no sensibility to pain or pleasure—no senses analogous, though inferior, to our own—no grateful sense of kindness, nor suffering from neglect or injury; if we discovered, in short, nothing but mere animated matter, obviously and exclusively sub-servient to human purposes, it would be difficult to maintain that the dominion over them was a trust, in any other sense, at least, than to make the best use for ourselves of the property in them which Providence had given us. But it calls for no deep or extended skill in natural history to know that the very reverse of this is the case, and that God is the benevolent and impartial author of all that He has created. For every animal which comes in contact with man, and whose powers and qualities and instincts are obviously adapted to his use, Nature has taken care to provide, and as carefully and bountifully as for man himself, organs and feelings for its own enjoyment and happiness. . . . The animals are given for our use, but not for our abuse. Their freedom and enjoyments, when they cease to be consistent with our just dominion and enjoyments, can be no part of their natural rights; but whilst they are consistent, their rights, subservient as they are, ought to be as sacred as our own."—*Speech of Lord Erskine in the House of Peers*, 1809.

MORPHIA. Bernard.

CLAUDE BERNARD (the late), M.D., Paris, Prof. Exper. Physiol. Coll. de France, 1855; Prof. Gen. Physiol. at Museum, 1868-78 (born 1813; died 1878). (V.)

"The dose that we ordinarily employ is one of 5 centi-grammes, but one may give to the dog without danger a stronger dose, even double the quantity, of morphia, provided the drug is perfectly pure. The animal still remains sensitive: a touch on the cornea induces the closing of the eyelids; but he lies quite still, and lends himself without a movement to the most delicate operations. . . .

"He feels the pain, but has lost the idea of self-defence."— *Leçons de Physiologie Opératoire*, by Claude Bernard (Paris, 1879), p. 155.

—— The same—Contradictory Effects of, Berdoe. on Animals and Man,

EDWARD BERDOE, M.R.C.S., L.R.C.P.Ed., London. (A.V.)

"'As regards man,' says Dr. Ringer (p. 494), 'morphia is the most powerful alkaloid [of opium]; but, according to Bernard, as regards animals it ranks fourth.'

❊   ❊   ❊   ❊   ❊

"Morphia is a powerful poison to man, a quarter of a grain

being an ordinary dose as a medicinal agent. Yet 'birds,' says Stillé, 'tolerate the action of morphia to an almost incredible degree.' A pigeon has been known to survive a dose of 12 grains."—*The Futility of Experiments with Drugs on Animals*, by Edward Berdoe (London, 1889), p. 30.

MOUNTAIN LAUREL (*Kalmia Latifolia*)   Berdoe.
Different Effect of, on Man and Animals.

EDWARD BERDOE, M.R.C.S., L.R.C.P.Ed., London.   (A.V.)

" The leaves and berries of this American plant are poisonous to man, but partridges feed on its berries, and their flesh kills men who eat it, as it acts upon them as a sedative poison. This was at one time doubted, and the physiologists thought that its poisonous action upon man must be due to putrefaction of the game. It was hard to have to admit that birds could eat berries which were poisonous to human beings, so Dr. Stabler tried a strong decoction of the plant upon himself, and found the fact was precisely as stated. An allied plant, *Andromeda Mariana*, is called 'stagger bush,' and is fatal to lambs and calves.—(*Stillé*, p. 798.)"—*The Futility of Experiments with Drugs on Animals*, by Edward Berdoe (London, 1889), p. 28.

MYXŒDEMA AND VIVISECTION.   Berdoe.

EDWARD BERDOE, M.R.C.S., L.R.C.P.Ed., London.   (A.V.)

" May I be permitted to point out, with reference to 'R. G.'s' note on myxœdema and vivisection, an important inaccuracy in his statement that a cure for this hideous disease has been discovered by vivisection ? When the thyroid gland is excised in the human being he becomes a cretin. Yet rabbits endure the operation well, and so do sheep, calves, and horses. Of dogs, cats, and foxes only a very few survive. Schiff found that, if one half of the gland was excised at once and the other half a month afterwards, death did not occur. Wagner denied this. Horsley made a number of investigations, and discovered that he could produce myxœdema, but was unable to cure it, and there is to this day no cure for the malady. Dr. Murray, of Newcastle, discovered, but not by vivisection, that an injection of the extract of the thyroid gland of a sheep into myxœdemic patients would avert death and improve the health of the patients; but the treatment must be persisted in regularly, or he relapses. I am informed by one who is himself a vivisector that certain animals in a laboratory from whom the thyroid gland had been removed, and who, in consequence, became very ill, suddenly improved in health in a manner which puzzled the experimenters till it was found that they had been eating a quantity of thyroid glands which had been thrown in a corner. I am told that this accident suggested the new treatment. . . . Where 'R. G.' is wrong is in stating that the disease can be cured by merely swallowing the thyroid tablet. Neither is it right to omit reference to King's researches in 1836. King showed that the thyroid secreted a peculiar fluid, which found entrance to the general system through the lymphatics. Afterwards Crede, Resas, Alberboni, and others, made researches in the same direction : and, though it is true that Horsley has made important contributions to our knowledge of the pathology of myxœdema, such means as we possess of averting death from the disease were bestowed upon humanity by Dr. Murray, who did not make his discovery by vivisection."—*Letter in the "Agnostic Journal,"* April 28th, 1894.

MYXŒDEMA AND VIVISECTION—Horsley   Murray. not the Originator of Thyroid Treatment.

GEORGE R. MURRAY, M.B.Camb., M.R.C.P.Lond., Newcastle-on-Tyne. (V.)

" It was found by Dr. von Eiselsberg that if the thyroid gland was successfully transplanted from the neck of an animal to some other part of the body, it was capable of continuing its functions, and so preventing the onset of the symptoms which would otherwise have followed its removal from the neck. Mr. Horsley then suggested that grafting a healthy sheep's thyroid gland into a patient suffering from myxœdema should be tried as a means of arresting the progress of the disease. This suggestion has since been carried out. . . . [Relates a case of treatment by injections of thyroid juice.] Many cases of myxœdema doubtless do improve to a certain extent when untreated, and it is not wise to draw many conclusions from a single case. . . . The improvement, of course, cannot be expected to be continued if the injections are discontinued, but there seems no reason why it should not be maintained if the injections are repeated at intervals of two or three weeks."—*British Medical Journal*, Oct. 18th, 1891, p. 796.

—— The same.   Clarke.

JOHN H. CLARKE, M.D., Physician to the Homœopathic Hospital, London. (A.V.)

" In Pepper's Medicine, vol. II., p. 242, I find it stated that

as early as 1873, Gull described cases of 'a cretinoid state
supervening in adult life in women.' In 1877 Dr. Ord
·grouped these cases under the term myxœdema, and discussed the relations of the condition to atrophy of the thyroid
gland, and to epidemic and sporadic cretinism. Kocher had
noticed that in certain instances of total extirpation of the
thyroid a remarkable cachexia is developed (*cachexia strumi-
priva*), which, in reality, is identical with the condition
described by Gull or Ord.' Where then was the necessity for
experiments on animals? They could only demonstrate (if
they demonstrated anything) facts already known. Even those
persons who need to be shown a rice pudding and a pound
of potatoes would hardly require this."—*Letter in* " *Weekly
Sun*," July 23rd, 1894.

MYXŒDEMA AND VIVISECTION—Horsley   Eulenburg.
not the Originator of Thyroid Treatment.

PROFESSOR EULENBURG, Berlin.   (P.V.)

" While agreeing fully with Prof. Ewald as to the beneficial
effects of the treatment of myxœdema with thyroid juice, I
may call to mind that American physicians have found that,
in general, these effects are not lasting, all the morbid symptoms reappearing directly the treatment is suspended."—*Debate
at Medical Society, Berlin, " Medical Week*," July 27th, 1894.

NEEDLESSNESS—The Royal College of
Veterinary Surgeons of Scotland on.

" The following protest is quoted by Sir William Fergusson :
· We, the Court of Examiners for Scotland of the Royal
College of Veterinary Surgeons, desire to express our opinion
that the performance of operations on living animals is
altogether unnecessary and useless for the purpose of causa-
tion. Signed, JAMES SYME, Chairman ; JAMES DUNSMORE,
President of the College of Surgeons of Edinburgh ; J.
WARBURTON BEGBIE, M.D. ; JOHN LAWSON, President of the
Royal College of Veterinary Surgeons; B. CARTLEDGE,
M.R.C.V.S., Member of Council of R.C.V.S. ; WILLIAM
COCKBURN, M.R.C.V.S.; WILLIAM ROBERTSON, M.R.C.V.S. ;
CHARLES SECKER, M.R.C.V.S. ; JAMES COWIE, M.R.C.V.S. I
fully concur in the above. JOHN WILKINSON, Principal
Veterinary Surgeon to the Forces."—*Roy. Com. Evidence*
(London, 1876), Q. 1,030.

NERVES, Sir C. Bell and the. Gimson.

W. GIMSON GIMSON, M.D., M.R.C.S., Witham, Essex. (A.V.)

" In pursuing his investigations, Sir Charles Bell was guided by anatomy, as he repeatedly informs us, and we find him evidently averse to *vivisection*, and only resorting to it to overthrow some pre-existing dogma, or to demonstrate his theories. Thus, in expounding his theory that the posterior roots were for sensation alone, it became as he thought necessary to overthrow the opinion which prevailed, that ganglia were intended to cut off sensation : or again, in demonstrating his idea of the analogy existing between the fifth nerve and the general system of spinal nerves, he made use of a few expeiiments, and some of those were upon animals recently killed."—*Vivisections and Painful Experiments on Living Animals : their Unjustifiability* (London, 1879), pp. 26, 27.

—— Bell's Discovery of the Uses of Roots Macaulay. of the Spinal.

JAMES MACAULAY, M.A., M.D., F.R.C.S.Ed., London. (A.V.)

" Next to the circulation of the blood, the discovery of the distinct offices of the anterior and posterior roots of the spinal nerves, and the columns from which they arise, is the favourite instance of the results of vivisection. It is strange how vivisectors insist on a claim which Sir Charles Bell has himself denied and repudiated. His express statements as to the purely anatomical source of his discovery have already been quoted. I have lately conversed on the subject with Mr. Shaw, Sir Charles Bell's friend and relative, and the able editor and expositor of his published researches. Mr. Shaw tells me that Sir Charles invariably spoke of his discovery as due to anatomical investigation ; that his experiments were performed with the utmost reluctance, and were considered by him unnecessary ; and that he often referred to the uselessness and cruelty of experiments on living animals. This is quite in accordance with the humane spirit that appears in all the writings of Sir Charles Bell."--*Vivisection, A Prize Essay* (London, 1881), p. 27.

—— The same.—Reflex Action of. Macaulay.

JAMES MACAULAY, M.A., M.D., F.R.C.S.Ed., London. (A.V.)

" Dr. Marshall Hall's discovery of reflex action, it is said, has led to great improvements in the treatment of epilepsy and other nervous diseases ; he discovered reflex action by experiments.   ✳   ✳   ✳   ✳   ✳

" The truth is that no experiments at all are needed for demon-strating the processes of reflex action, nor do they help towards applying the knowledge to practice, although this assertion is made. So far from leading to improved treatment of epilepsy, or other diseases supposed to be chiefly dependent on the spinal cord, the ill-digested knowledge of what Marshall Hall really did and taught has led to stupid routine, and contracted views of maladies which require most intelligent and varied treatment. This depends, in every individual case, upon con-ditions only to be ascertained by careful observation, or what Marshall Hall himself calls ' living pathology.' "—*Vivisection, A Prize Essay* (London, 1881), pp. 38, 39.

NERVES—Experiments on the, cannot be done under Anæsthetics.   Sharpey.

WILLIAM SHARPEY (the late), M.D., LL.D., F.R.S., formerly Professor of Physiology in University College (born 1802 ; died 1880). (V.)

" There is one point upon which I did not quite apprehend the difference of your answers. You stated early in your evi-dence that you thought a repetition of Sir Charles Bell's experi-ments would not be justifiable ; that where the facts have been successfully ascertained the experiments could not justifiably be used in the teaching of classes ?—No ; because in the first place they could not be used under anæsthetics. You see anæsthetics would destroy the sensibility, and you could not use such an experiment under anæsthetics. And it is a painful experiment in two ways : in the first place, exposing the spinal cord and laying bare the roots of the nerve is a very painful operation ; and that part of it might be done under anæsthe-tics, and then the animal may recover its sensibility ; but the subsequent prolongation of the experiment would be painful."—*Evid. Roy. Com.* (London, 1876), Q. 464.

NERVOUS SYSTEM, The, A Barrier to Man's Inquisitiveness.   Gimson.

W. GIMSON GIMSON, M.D., M.R.C.S., Witham, Essex. (A.V.)

" Bernard tells us that ' an operation performed on *a single point* of the nervous system gives rise (*in one instance*) to a general hyperæsthesia (or exalted sensation) of the *whole* apparatus.' In truth, the influence of that part of the nervous system which regulates the nutrition and function of every portion of the body, must ever be a barrier to man's inquisitiveness, and will ever prevent him reducing to scientific data those impenetrable agencies which govern and maintain life. To understand the laws which regulate the nervous system is beyond our power ; how then are we to analyze our disturbance of them ? "—*Vivisections and Painful Experiments on Living Animals : their Unjustifiability* (London, 1879), pp. 60, 61.

NITRITE OF AMYL.   Harris.

STANFORD HARRIS, M.R.C.S., L.S.A., London.   (A.V.)

" The facts of the discovery of nitrite of amyl are these : The French chemist Balard discovered the drug in 1844. In 1865, Dr. Richardson introduced it to the notice of the profession, and Dr. Gamgee afterwards made the experiments which Dr. Lauder Brunton says 'made me acquainted with its action,' and adds 'had it not been for those experiments we should, I think, still have been without a remedy for angina pectoris.'

" Now the action of nitrite of amyl is so obvious and immediate that no chemist or physician, who has ever held a bottle in his hand, can have failed to have had its effects demonstrated upon his face.   Directly one smells the vapour, the face flushes, and the arteries of the head expand and throb. According to Dr. Brunton, he arrived by observation of patients at the conclusion that 'the pain was actually caused by the rise of blood pressure in the vessels.'   Dr. Gamgee's experiments on animals proved that nitrite of amyl 'lessened the blood pressure in the vessels '—in plain words, dilates, flushes them.   Dr. Brunton deliberately chooses to go by the experiments on the animal rather than the numberless ones which must have continually occurred—as it were by accident —on all who ever handled the drug during the twenty years or more that it was handled, prior to these experiments.

    *   *   *   *   *

" To summarize : amyl nitrite was introduced by Dr. Richardson in 1865.   The experiments of Dr. Gamgee some years later are claimed as the foundation of its use in medicine.   It relieves, but does not cure, certain cases of angina pectoris, or spasm of the heart.   No one can handle a bottle of nitrite of amyl for two minutes without having its effects demonstrated upon his own face.   It dilates the blood vessels.   This fact could not fail to be known to each physician to whose notice Dr. Richardson had introduced it previous to Dr. Gamgee's experiments.   When Dr. Lauder Brunton was looking out for a dilator of the blood vessels to relieve angina pectoris, here was one to his hand.   In the words of Dr. McCormick,

N

Deputy-Inspector of H.M. Hospitals and Fleet, and of Arctic fame: 'The fact that amyl nitrite often relieves angina pectoris could have been very readily arrived at by letting a patient inhale its vapour. Animal torture was unnecessary.'"
—*Extracts from a Letter of Stanford Harris, M.R.C.S.*, 1888.

NITRITE OF AMYL. Brunton.

THOMAS LAUDER BRUNTON, M.D., D.Sc., F.R.S., Assistant Physician and Lecturer on Materia Medica at St. Bartholomew's Hospital, London, etc. (V.)

" Take the use of nitrite of amyl in certain forms of angina pectoris. The obvious symptoms in this disease are intense pain in the region of the heart, and fear of impending death. Sphygmographic tracings of the pulse, taken during this condition, show that the tension within the heart and vessels begins to increase as the pain comes on, and reaches such a height that the heart can barely empty itself. Observations on animals have shown that nitrite of amyl lessens the tension of the blood in the vessels ; and we therefore give it in angina pectoris with the expectation that it will diminish the tension and remove the pain, and we find that it succeeds."—*From " A Textbook of Pharmacology, Therapeutics, and Materia Medica,"* by T. L. Brunton (London, 1885), p. 2.

" Dr. Lauder Brunton said that after discovering the utility of nitrite of amyl many years ago. he went to work with Professor Ludwig in his laboratory at Leipzig, and there made further researches. He regretted to say, however, that he had been somewhat in the position of Solomon's sluggard, who would not roast his game after he had brought it home. He took the trouble to make a great number of experiments ; but he had not published them, and he had kept them to himself ever since 1869,[*] always thinking that he would have something more to add to perfect them, and he had never got them out until now. At that time he made some experiments with nitrite of ethyl and with nitrite of sodium, and found that both these nitrites lowered the blood pressure. He thus satisfied himself that the action upon the blood-pressure was not due to the amyl, but was due to the salt employed being a nitrite. Some years later, in 1876, he asked Mr. Gresswell to engage with him in researches upon the action of various nitrites and they tested the effect of the nitrite of ethyl, the nitrite of propyl, and the nitrite of capryl in comparison with the action of nitrite of amyl. The results had only been mentioned in the

---

[*] Dr. B. W. Richardson introduced it to the profession in 1865. See above.

St. Bartholomew's Hospital Reports, and had not been published in any other way. They found that the nitrite of amyl appeared to differ from the other nitrites in possessing a very much more active power to dilate the vessels and to lower the blood-pressure. All those experiments were open to the objection that the substances with which they experimented were not chemically pure. He wished to point out that the nitrite of amyl, so-called, as purchased in the shops, varied in the effects it produced to a very considerable extent. The pure nitrite of amyl did not produce such a marked action as the commercial specimen; but in all probability the explanation of that was given by Professor Cash, who found that butyl nitrite was the more powerful of the two, and probably the commercial article contained a large percentage of that."— *Speech printed in "British Medical Journal,"* Jan. 5th, 1889.

NITRITE OF AMYL AND ANGINA PECTORIS. Leech.

D. J. LEECH, M.D., Professor of Materia Medica, Owen's College Manchester. (P.V.)

" The inhalation of amyl nitrite sometimes fails to relieve the pain of angina pectoris ; this failure may arise from several causes :—

" 1. The paroxysms may be due to neuralgia of local origin, or it may be reflected or hysterical, and circulatory changes may take but little part in its production. In such conditions nitrite inhalations can do no harm, yet they may fail to relieve pain.

" 2. In some cases the nitrite does not remove pain because of the short duration of its action. It does not break the spell of the vessel contraction. There may be relief, but it is not complete, and when in a minute or two the effect of the drug passes off the wave of contraction returns, and with it the pain.

" 3. Some persons are curiously insusceptible to the influence of amyl nitrite. In such patients full inhalations may succeed when slight ones fail, though this is not very common. If a certain measure of success is not obtained with ordinary inhalation, it is not often that a more copious use of amyl nitrite completely removes anginal pain.

" 4. Lastly, in very advanced cases where the attacks of pain continue long, amyl nitrite may entirely fail to relieve the pain, though in an earlier stage it proved useful for this purpose."—*Croonian Lecture on " The Nitrates and Allied Compounds," "Lancet,"* July 15th, 1893, p. 124.

" SYNCOPE AND CARDIAC FAILURE.—The difficulty is to graduate the amount of nitrite to the necessities of the heart. If any nitrite were, by inhalation, thrown into the blood in large quantities it might stop the action of a failing heart."—*Ibid*, p. 126.

" MIGRAINE AND HEADACHE.—The drug, indeed, has not maintained its promise; the utility attributed to it in the account of earlier reporters has not been borne out by frequent experience."—*Ibid*, p. 127.

NORWICH EXPERIMENTS, THE.   Magnan. (V.)

[In August, 1874, during the Congress of the British Medical Association, Dr. Magnan, at the Masonic Hall, Norwich, experimented on a dog by injecting alcohol and absinthe into the veins and blood-vessels. A prosecution afterwards instituted on a charge of cruelty ended fruitlessly. The following extracts, laid before the Royal Commission in 1875, are here inserted as evidence of what the experiments involved, the descriptions being by Dr. Magnan himself.]

" If one continues to administer a daily dose of alcohol sufficient to bring on intoxication, one remarks in the dog from about the fifteenth day a nervous excitability of quite peculiar character. The animal is melancholy and uneasy : he listens, the least noise makes him start ; when the door is opened, seized with fright he runs and crouches in the darkest corner of the room ; he no longer responds when patted, he runs away and tries to bite when one attempts to take hold of him, and utters sharp cries at the mere threat of blows. This irritable and timid condition increases each day, and from the end of the first month, illusions and hallucinations becoming added to it, it is transformed into a veritable delirium. In the middle of the night he utters plaintive moans, or even whilst all is quiet he begins to bark, the cries becoming louder and more frequent as if an enemy were approaching ; speaking or calling does not reassure him, one must interfere with a light. At last, during the day he growls without cause ; then, thinking that he is pursued, he cries out, runs scared hither and thither, with his head turned back and snapping in the air."—*Dr. Magnan*, " *The Lancet*," No. 2,664 p. 411.

" What we see in the dog, in some cases, after intravenous, subcutaneous, or stomachical injections of essence of absinthe is as follows :—In the interval between two epileptic attacks, and sometimes before the convulsive symptoms, or even without convulsions, the animal is seized with an attack of delirium.

All of a sudden he erects himself on his paws, the hair bristles, the look becomes wild, the eyes injected and brilliant, staring at some particular spot where there is nothing apparent to draw his attention ; he barks furiously, advances and retires as before an enemy, with open mouth he throws his head suddenly forwards, and immediately shuts his jaws and shakes them from side to side, as if he wished to tear his prey in pieces. This attack of delirium may recur several times ; then the effects pass off, and the animal becomes quite calm."—*Dr. Magnan*, " *The Lancet*," No. 2,664, p. 411.

NORWICH EXPERIMENTS, THE.   Taylor.

ALFRED SWAYNE TAYLOR (the late), M.D., F.R.C.P. (born 1806 ; died 1880). (A.V.)

" Were you at. all aware what passed at Norwich when a great deal of attention was drawn to the subject ?—I read in the medical journals what did pass about some injections that were made into a dog. To me they appeared to be of a most cruel kind, and to answer no purpose justifying the nature of the experiment."—*Evid. Roy. Com.* (London, 1876), Q. 1,188.

NUMBER OF VIVISECTIONS Performed.   Harris.

STANFORD HARRIS, M.R.C.S., London. (A.V.)

That the number, however, of victims to vivisection is likely to be much greater than is generally supposed may be inferred from such facts as the following :—

Q. 994 : A paper (read by Mr. Hutton) by Brown-Séquard, in which he described himself as having " at one time before the siege of Paris 584 guinea-pigs in my laboratory," and added " I can say I have had many and many thousands under observation from 1843 till now, a period of more than thirty years." (For the nature of these very painful experiments see page 377, appendix iv., of Blue Book.) At Q. 5,747 Dr. Brunton says : " When I said ninety I should have said that was in one series. I used a much larger number." Q. 5,748 : " For the snake poison experiments I should think I have used about 150 of ' all sorts '—rabbits, guinea-pigs, frogs, dogs, pigeons, and fowls." Q. 3,361 : Dr. Ferrier spoke of 100 animals being vivisected by him previous to a certain date.

A report of a lecture given by M. Flourens records (Blatin *Nos Cruautés*, pp. 201, 202) the experimentations of himself and Majendie to establish the distinctions of the sensory and the motor nerves, according to Sir Charles Bell, upon over 8,000 dogs.

Monsieur Pasteur inoculates the brains of two rabbits per diem with rabies, if the account in the *Nineteenth Century* of June, 1888, by an admirer may be taken as evidence.— "*Darwin and the Royal Commission*," by S. Harris (1888).

NUMBER OF VIVISECTIONS Performed.   Bell.

ERNEST BELL, M.A., London.   (A.V.)

1st. The number of licensed vivisectors has increased (according to the Parliamentary Returns) from twenty-three in 1876 to 184 in 1893. This last number does not, however, represent the actual number of persons engaged in vivisection, as assistants are frequently employed who hold no licenses ; and in three cases in which experiments have been reported in the medical papers as made by a man who was unlicensed, the Victoria Street Society, on appealing to the Home Secretary, has received the answer that the report was incorrect, the gentleman named not having done the operations himself, but having only assisted Professor So-and-So, who held a license. It will be seen that by this method one license may be made to cover a multitude of sinners.

2nd. During the same period the number of licensed places has increased from 19 to 56 ; the total number of experiments has risen from 481 to 4,046, and those performed wholly, or in part, without anæsthetics from 117 to 2,845. Nor can *these* figures be accepted as giving the whole increase, as in several important cases it has been shown that experiments published in scientific journals have not been included in the Returns, and the presumption is great that others have been omitted in the same way.

3rd. The fact that there has existed for some years in Cambridge a " Scientific Instrument Company," which provides the appliances needed for vivisection, is strong evidence that there must be a good demand for such tools, some of which being very costly (from £20 to £60), would certainly not be kept in stock unless they were frequently purchased. In the catalogue we find amongst others the following items :—Artificial Respiration Apparatus ("suitable to the largest dog or the smallest rabbit"), Batteries, Cannulæ, Catheters, Clamps, Dog-holders ("improved from Bernard's model and suited for both large and small animals"), Onkometer ("Roy's, in two sizes, for the kidney of the rabbit and dog"), Onkometer ("Roy's, in two sizes, for spleen of dog"), Plethysmograph ("Roy's, for the leg of the dog"), Rabbit-holder ("modified from Czermak's form," etc.), Tetanus spring ("the number of stimulations per second of the nerve may be raised to any extent required," etc.), Universal Holders (" Roy's "). Another large establishment for the sale of similar instruments is Messrs. Hawksley, Oxford Street, London.

4th. Practical physiology has been endowed of late years in a marked degree.

In 1879 was founded the G. H. Lewes scholarship (value £200 a year) for physiological research, by the aid of which Professor Roy was enabled to perform the agonising experiments which were quoted by Mr. Reid in the House of Commons.

In 1884 the University of Oxford voted £10,000 for the erection of a laboratory for Professor Burdon-Sanderson, editor and joint author of the manual which was one of the immediate causes of the appointment of the Royal Commission. It was on account of this vote on the part of his University that Professor Ruskin felt called upon to resign his professorship.

In 1887 another sum of £10,000 was left by Mr. J. Lucas Walker for the purposes of scientific and literary research. The then Attorney-General (Sir R. Webster), into whose hands the bequest was committed, acting on the advice of three friends well known for their advocacy and practice of vivisection, determined to found with it a studentship for experimental pathology, the holder of which is to be under the immediate control of Professor Roy.

In 1887 also, Sir Erasmus Wilson having bequeathed upwards of £200,000 to the Royal College of Surgeons for the benefit of their College, there appeared in the *British Medical Journal* of January 15th, a Round-robin addressed to the President, Vice-Presidents, and Council of the College, praying that a portion of this sum might be devoted to the erection of an institution like the " splendid laboratories " of Berlin, Paris, Leipzig, etc. Of the fifty-two scientific men by whom this memorial was signed, thirty one, at least, had either actually practised vivisection or publicly advocated the practice, and demanded the repeal of the present law ; and nineteen of them had held licenses, of whom seventeen had the additional certificate dispensing with the necessity for keeping the animals unconscious of their sufferings. Fortunately, the Protest of the Victoria Street Society with 40,000 signatures stopped the scheme for a time, but it would appear that the Council of the College of Surgeons have since endowed the Pathological Laboratories on the Victoria Embankment.— (*See letter of Dr. Rutter in "Stciz," Aug. 13th, 1891.*)

In 1887 the College of Physicians of Edinburgh voted the sum of £1,000 for the establishment of a Research Laboratory, and, further, one-third of their surplus annual income for its maintenance.

In 1887 the Senate of the University of Cambridge gave their sanction to the preparation of plans for a Physiological Laboratory, the cost of which was estimated at £10,000. In part execution of this plan Dr. Sidgwick, Professor of Moral Philosophy in the University, made an offer of £1,500 as a contribution to the expense of the proposed new buildings for the Department of Physiology, provided that the buildings were proceeded with at once. Accordingly, by grace of the Senate, carried by thirteen votes against five on the 21st November, 1889, not only was Dr. Sidgwick's offer accepted with thanks, but a further sum of £3,500 was voted for the erection of the new buildings, which were proceeded with accordingly.

In 1890 an appeal was made in the *Times* by the committee of the Brown Institution for additional funds. The institution, originally founded for the benefit of animals, by a benevolent man, who expressly stated : " I further desire that kindness to animals committed to its charge shall be the general principle of the institution," has since fallen into the hands of the physiologists, who, with Victor Horsley at their head, and eleven licensed vivisectors under him, have used it as a vivisection laboratory at their discretion. The exact amount collected from the appeal has apparently not been announced, but a list of subscriptions was published, including those of four of the City companies.

In 1891 we had before us two important and significant appeals of a similar nature. One at Cambridge, for the foundation of an institute similar to the Pasteur Institute at Paris. The executive committee consisted of five licensed vivisectors and two ardent advocates of the practice, one of whom promised £500 conditionally, while other sums were subscribed.

The second appeal was for £50,000 for the endowment of " modern science and experimental research" at King's College, London. With regard to this it may be mentioned that Lord Chief Justice Coleridge refused to append his signature to the appeal, because the promoters would not give their assurance that experiments on living animals would not be included in their "experimental research."

It cannot be too strongly impressed on the public that vivisection is not an occasional practice resorted to only in special cases to settle some disputed points. It is on the contrary an organized and systematized *method*—a method which the Royal Commission pronounced as " from its very nature liable to great abuse," and, so long as this method is sanctioned at all, it will have a constant tendency to increase, as Professor Lankester said, "in something like geometrical ratio."—*From "Vivisection on the Increase."* By Ernest Bell (London, 1891), pp. 1–4.

OBSERVATION, without Experiments, would suffice. Cuvier.

GEORGES CUVIER, Author of the well-known Work on Natural History (born 1769 ; died 1852). (A.V.)

" Nature has supplied the opportunities of learning that which experiments on the living body never could furnish. It presents us, in the different classes of animals, with nearly all possible combinations of organs, and in all proportions. There are none but have some description of organs by which they are made familiar to us ; and it only is needful to examine closely the effects produced by these combinations, and the results of their partial or total absence, to deduce very probable conclusions as to the nature and use of each organ, and of each form of organ in man."—*Letter to J. C. Mertrud, Prof. of Animal Anatomy, Nat. Hist. Museum, Paris,* in " *Leçons d'Anatomie Comparée* " (1835).

OPIUM. Berdoe.

EDWARD BERDOE, M.R.C.S., L.R.C.P.Ed., London. (A.V.)

" Let us imagine that a quantity of a new drug, called opium, is being examined for the first time.

*   *   *   *   *

" The physiologists proceed to investigate its action by a long series of experiments upon animals ; they give it to frogs, and they find that small doses throw them into tetanic spasms. Next they try it on a pigeon, to which they give twenty grains, and it is none the worse for it. Emboldened by their success, they give thirty grains to a rabbit, and no effect is produced. They discover that ducks and chickens, like the pigeons and rabbits, are never the worse for its administration. They resolve now to try it on a hospital patient, and proceeding with extreme caution, as they think, they decide not to venture at first beyond the dose they gave to the pigeon, namely, twenty grains. The patient is a powerful navvy, yet to their consternation and distress he is promptly killed by the dose. If physiological medicine were of any value, surely the method followed by these investigators was right and cautious. Yet how fatal their method when reduced to practice. When opium is administered to human beings in large doses it contracts the pupils to a pin point; in birds the pupils are not affected; in horses they are widely dilated; in dogs under its influence the pupils first dilate and then contract. Opium seems as if it were created to confound the physiologists. Dr. Mitchell says it is impossible to kill a pigeon by opium given by the mouth; but Flourens affirms that a single grain will throw a sparrow into profound stupor. None of the opium preparations cause sleep in pigeons, ducks, or chickens. With dogs, cats, and rabbits large doses of opium produce sleep, usually with convulsions. In frogs opium only causes tetanus. Race greatly modifies its effects on man. It drives Javanese and Malays into temporary madness. (*Ringer*, *Materia Medica*, 5th Ed., p. 478)."—*The Futility of Experiments with Drugs on Animals*, by Edward Berdoe (London, 1889), pp. 29, 30.

OVARIOTOMY. Magee.

RIGHT REV. W. G. MAGEE (the late), Bishop of Peterborough, and afterwards Archbishop of York (born 1821; died 1891). (P.V.)

" A London medical man of the highest eminence* owes a discovery by which he has saved hundreds of lives to a series of experiments performed upon a dozen rabbits."—*Bishop of Peterborough's Speech, House of Lords*, July 15th, 1879.

—— The same. Wells.

SIR SPENCER WELLS, Bart., London; Hon. F.R.C.S., 1844; M., 1841; F.R.C.P.I. (Hon.), 1867; late Prof. of Surg. and Path., R.C.S., Eng. (V.)

" If we could hope in diseased women for the same series of changes as have been observed in healthy dogs and rabbits, we might agree more completely with the conclusions of the German experimenters. But it is one thing to remove a piece of a uterine horn, or a healthy ovary, or a bit of omentum or mesentery, from a dog or a rabbit, and a very different thing to remove a large uterine or ovarian tumour from a woman whose

---

* Sir Spencer Wells is here referred to, together with his operation in abdominal surgery, commonly called " Ovariotomy." (*See* Ovariotomy—WELLS.)

general health has been more or less affected by the growth of the tumour."—*Diseases of the Ovaries*, by Sir S. Wells (London. 1872), p. 372.

OVARIOTOMY—The First Successful Performance of.   Wells.

SIR SPENCER WELLS, F.R.C.S., F.R.C.P.I., M.D., F.R.C.S.I., London. (V.)

" No one can dispute the validity of the direct claim of McDowell* as practically the first successful ovariotomist. . . . He lost only the last of his first five cases of ovariotomy, and thus as it were established at the outset what until recently was complacently regarded as a satisfactory standard of mortality for so serious an operation."—*On Ovarian and Uterine Tumours, their Diagnosis and Treatment*, by T. Spencer Wells (London, 1882), pp. 184-5.

—— The same—Wells' First Case.   Wells.

SIR SPENCER WELLS, F.R.C.S., F.R.C.P.I., M.D., F.R.C.S.I., London. (V.)

" During the autumn of 1857, a young woman was under treatment [at the Samaritan Hospital] for what appeared to be an ovarian tumour on the left side. . . . I determined to see what it was, and in December, 1857, twenty-four years ago, I prepared for my first ovariotomy. . . . As soon as I opened the peritoneum, and it was proved beyond all doubt that the tumour was behind the intestines, I was induced very unwillingly to close the wound, and do nothing more."—*On Ovarian and Uterine Tumours, their Diagnosis and Treatment*, by T. Spencer Wells (London, 1882), p. 196.

—— The same—Wells sees Clay operate.   Clay.

CHARLES CLAY, M.D. (the late), Manchester (born 1801 ; died 1893). (A.V.)

" Fifteen years after my first operation (in 1842), Mr. S. Wells came to Manchester to be present at one of my operations, and made many enquiries, amongst which—'Did I include the peritoneum in my interrupted sutures ?' I replied, 'Certainly ;' and gave as my reason, that in two cases where the suture had not included the peritoneum hernial protrusions had followed.

* Dr. Ephraim McDowell, a Virginian, practising in Kentucky, who had studied under John Bell, in Edinburgh, in 1794. He died in 1814, aged 78.—*Wells*.

I also added, that peritonitis could only be set up *once*, whether
the sutures included the peritoneum or not. I was for some
time after in correspondence with Mr. Wells, but never heard
of vivisection in connection with ovariotomy, nor can I perceive any advantage that ovariotomy has received from such
experiments. All my operations from first to last have shown
the same average amount of success—about 75 per cent. I
have never practised nor yet countenanced vivisection. I have
given up operating after 400 cases and about 100 deaths."—
Letter of Dr. Clay, dated April 6th, 1880.

OVARIOTOMY—Wells sees Clay operate.   Clay,

CHARLES CLAY, M.D. (the late), Manchester (born 1801 ; died
       1893). (A.V.)

" I have lived to see ovariotomy established as an operation
years before Mr. S. Wells ever operated. . . . You state
that Mr. Wells took great care to include the peritoneum in
the sutures uniting the abdominal wound—a practice based on
scientific experimental evidence. This has always been my
practice since my first case in 1842, fifteen years before Mr.
Wells ever operated at all, and was the advice given to him
when he visited me."—*Letter signed* CHARLES CLAY, M.D.,
British Medical Journal, July 3rd, 1880, p. 32.

—— The same.   Clay.

CHARLES CLAY, M.D. (the late), Manchester (born 1801 ; died
       1893). (A.V.)

" You say, ' We are informed that Mr. Wells never saw Dr.
Clay operate before he operated himself, and only once some
years after his (Mr. Wells') first case.' In answer to this gross
and unpardonable misrepresentation,with Mr. Wells' admission
that his first case was in 1858 (his visit to me was in 1857),
will he deny, when confronted with two other gentlemen also
present, who heard him declare how much gratified he was to
see the operation for the first time, and who heard the number
of inquiries he made concerning it—will Mr. Wells deny his
own letter of thanks to me afterwards ? "—*Letter signed*
CHARLES CLAY, M.D., *British Medical Journal*, July 17th, 1880,
pp. 109-10.

—— The same—Vivisection no connection with,   Clay.

CHARLES CLAY, M.D., (the late), Manchester (born 1801 ; died
       1893). (A.V.)

" In my opinion vivisection has no more to do with advanc-

ing the success of ovariotomy than the Pope at Rome."—
Letter signed CHARLES CLAY, in *British Medical Journal*, July
17th, 1880, p. 110.

OVARIOTOMY—Vivisection no connection with.   Keith.

THOMAS KEITH, M.D.Ed., F.R.C.S.Ed., Edinburgh.   (V.)

" As to the other point of Dr. Clay's letter, of which so much
has lately been written—the uniting of the peritoneal surfaces*
   * The point as to which Mr. S. Wells' experiments on animals were made.
in closing the wound—little or no importance need be attached
to it as affecting the mortality."—*Letter of* THOMAS KEITH in
British Medical Journal, July 31st, 1880.

—— The same.   Simpson.

SIR JAMES SIMPSON (the late), Edinburgh (born 1811 ; died
   1870. (P.V.)

" My dear Dr. Clay—The operation is your own ; none can
rob you of your claim. Call it ovariotomy, not peritoneal
section. Your success is brilliant."—*Letter to* DR. CLAY, 1847.

—— The same.   Tait.

LAWSON TAIT, F.R.C.S., late Professor of Gynæcology, Queen's
   College, Birmingham. (A.V.)

" I have exhaustively studied the history of this operation,
since its first successful performance by Robert Houston in
1701. Its history may be divided, roughly speaking, into three
phases. The first begins with Ephraim McDowel, and ends
with Nathan Smith about the year 1824 ; and, during these
years, the whole achievements of modern surgery were almost
equalled in success, if not in extent. The principle of the
intraperitoneal treatment of the pedicle with the short ligature
was fully established : and the great regret. in the history of
the operation, is that it was ever departed from. The second
phase begins with Charles Clay, who first performed ovariotomy
in England on September 27th, 1842 ; and during the succeeding twenty-five years he performed 390 ovariotomies, with a
mortality of very nearly 25 per cent. This second phase ends
with the close of the career of Mr. Baker Brown in 1867. Dr.
Charles Clay, unfortunately, departed from the principles of
Nathan Smith, and used long ligatures. Baker Brown, on the
other hand, adopted a complete intraperitoneal method ; and
between May, 1855, and September, 1867, he performed 40

consecutive operations upon this principle, with a mortality of only 10 per cent. The third phase in the history of ovariotomy begins with Mr. Spencer Wells, who, between 1857 and 1878, performed 1,000 ovariotomies, with a mortality of 25 per cent.; he having, most unfortunately, like his predecessor, Dr. Clay, departed from the successful method of Nathan Smith. This third phase ends with Dr. Thomas Keith, who again re-established Nathan Smith's principle; and from that, I venture to say, no one will ever again have the hardihood to make a deviation. With this simple statement of the facts of the case it is difficult to see upon what basis your claim for Sir Spencer Wells is founded."—Letter in *British Medical Journal*, May 29th, 1886.*

OVARIOTOMY.   Tait.

LAWSON TAIT, F.R.C.S., late Professor of Gynæcology, Queen's
   College, Birmingham.   (A.V.)

"Disregarding all the conclusions of experiment, Baker Brown showed us how to bring our mortality of ovariotomy down to 10 per cent. ; and again in 1876, Keith proved that it might be still further reduced. The method of this reduction were such as only experience on human patients could indicate ; experiments on animals could and did teach nothing, for operations have been performed on thousands of animals every year for centuries, and nothing whatever has been learnt from this wholesale vivisection."—*Uselessness of Vivisection*, p. 17.

—— The same.   Bowie.

JOHN BOWIE, L.R.C.P., L.R.C.S., Edinburgh.   (A.V.)

"This operation [ovariotomy] has of late been prominently pushed forward as one of the trophies of vivisection. We are glad, however, to be able to state that the author of the operation positively disclaims any indebtedness to experiments on animals as either suggesting the operation itself or any modification of its performance. To Dr. Keith, of this city [Edinburgh], anti-vivisectionists owe a debt of gratitude for the

---

* Sir S. Wells claimed to have saved 500 lives at the cost of experiments on fourteen rabbits; but Mr. Lawson Tait has reduced the mortality after the operation of ovariotomy far below that of Sir S. Wells—to *nil*, in fact—without reference to any vivisection at all ; and Dr. Chas. Clay, who successfully performed the operation long before Sir S. Wells attempted it, testified that vivisection had "no more to do with ovariotomy than the Pope at Rome."—(See *Ovariotomy*—CLAY—*ante.*)

noble testimony he gave in the *British Medical Journal* of July, 1880, in repudiating the alleged results of Mr. Spencer Wells' experiments on rabbits in diminishing the number of deaths following the operation of ovariotomy.

   *   *   *   *   *

" To Dr. Charles Clay, of Manchester, belongs the honour of having first introduced into surgical practice the operation of ovariotomy. Through a long series of difficulties and discouragements he has given the medical profession an example of perseverance and assiduity in the pursuit of surgical science which few have equalled, and certainly none have surpassed." —*Reply to Dr. Rutherford*, Dec. 24th, 1880 (*Review* Office, 20, St. Giles Street, Edinburgh), p. 28.

PAIN—Admission as to Consciousness to.   Ferrier.

DAVID FERRIER, M.D., F.R.S., Professor of Neuropathy, King's College, London. (V.)

Dr. Ferrier, examined as to the experiment performed by him on monkeys, stated to be entirely under anæsthetics, in answer to Question 3,364 says, " I think I saw no indications of the animal suffering pain." (3,365) : " But you have expressed yourself so in this article as to many cases. At page 79, for instance, 'Experimental Researches in Cerebral Physiology and Pathology in the West Riding Lunatic Asylum Medical Reports,' I see you say, ' In order to determine whether the combined movements were conditioned by the voluntary impulse of the left hemisphere, I next proceeded, two hours after the removal of the right hemisphere, to expose the sigmoid gyrus of the superior external convolution of the left hemisphere. Having ascertained by electrisation that I could induce the usual movements of the right foreleg by stimulation of its centres here situated, I cut away the greater part of this gyrus, checking the hæmorrhage with cotton wool steeped in perchloride of iron. After this the animal ceased to struggle, and lay in whatever position it was placed. Pinching the toes caused reflex movements in all the four limbs, and at the same time the animal barked energetically, and howled when pinched. Pinching the tail especially caused the animal to bark. This condition continued for several hours, barking being always elicited and some reflex movements of the legs, but not to any great extent. The barking may also have been a reflex phenomenon, but from the fact that barking alone was sometimes induced, without any marked reflex movements of the limbs, I was rather inclined to attribute the phenomenon

to retention of consciousness and distinct sense of pain. Ultimately (five hours after the operation) no barking was caused,
but only reflex of the limbs and trunk when the legs or tail were
pinched. The dog survived for eight hours after the removal
of the hemispheres.' In that case clearly you did believe that
the animal was suffering."—"My last answer was with
reference to the experiments on the electrical excitation of the
brain, and that one which you have now read I had not in my
mind ; and even there I had very considerable difficulty in
determining whether the animal was conscious or not." (3,366):
"Still your opinion was that it was conscious ?"—"That was
the opinion to which I came in the end."—*Evid. Roy. Com.*
(London, 1876).

PAIN—Experiments have not mitigated.   Fergusson.

SIR WILLIAM FERGUSSON, BART., F.R.S. (the late), Surgeon
   to King's College Hospital, Sergeant Surgeon to the Queen,
   (born 1808 ; died 1877). (A.V.)

   " You have stated that you consider that experiments involving cruelty to animals have been too frequent, and that they
have not led to the mitigation of pain, generally speaking ; but
I presume you did not mean to say that they have not led to the
successful treatment of complaints, or the mitigation of human
suffering at all ?—With reference to that I may perhaps speak
more confidently regarding surgery than other departments in
my own profession, and in surgery I am not aware of any of
these experiments on the lower animals having led to the
mitigation of pain or to improvement as regards surgical
details."—*Evid. Roy. Com.* (London, 1876), Q. 1,049.

—— The same—A Good Motive no   Macaulay.
Excuse for the Infliction of.

JAMES MACAULAY, M.A., M.D., F.R.C.S.Ed., London.   (A.V.)

   " Except for self-defence or self-preservation, the moral sense
recoils from the infliction of pain and injury, even when a lofty
motive may be urged. Why has trial by torture been banished
from the jurisprudence of every civilised nation ? The object
of the rack and the thumbscrew, and of all the infernal apparatus in use in our courts of law at no very remote period, was
not to cause pain, far less to give any satisfaction or pleasure.
The discovery of truth was the object in this method of inter-
rogation ; and with this end in view, the use of torture was
justified, and directed by rulers and judges in other respects

humane as well as just. In the still more horrible tortures of the Inquisition, the object was not avowedly that of vindictive punishment ; nor need we assume that even the lowest executioners and officers of that dark tribunal took pleasure in the agonies of their heretic victims. The professed aim was higher even than in the processes of ordinary torture in courts of law. The advancement of Divine truth and of sacred science, or theology, was the alleged design of the Inquisition, while the spiritual welfare and eternal salvation of men might be also attained, through subjecting them to short though sharp affliction. Yet examination by torture is advocated by no one, because the infliction of pain, even for the advancement of truth, is not justifiable."—*Vivisection, A Prize Essay* (London, 1881), pp. 76, 77.

PAIN—Deliberate Infliction of, on Animals. Mantegazza.

PAOLO MANTEGAZZA, Professor of Pathology at the University of Pavia. (V.)

" The *Gazetta Italiana di Milano* contains an essay of Prof. Mantegazza on experiments carried on under his direction at the laboratory of experimental pathology of the University of Pavia. It will suffice to state that the experiments were intended to study the action of pain on digestion and nutrition. They were, as the Professor himself confesses, agonising to the animals subjected to them, and distressing to the experimenters, and simply proved that loss of appetite, great weakness, and a peculiar imbibition of moisture were the result of the pain inflicted. It is added that no alteration of the spinal marrow could be detected after the agony had been protracted for *one month*. Very meagre results of unpardonable cruelty."—*The Lancet* (March 25th, 1871), p. 415.

—— The same—Pathetic Incident in a Laboratory. Clarke.

JOHN H. CLARKE, M.D., Physician to the Homœopathic Hospital, London, S.W. (A.V.)

" Your well-known love for animals encourages me to hope you will find room for an account of one of the most touching incidents of animal affection ever recorded. The account is to be found in an article by C. Egerton Jennings, F.R.C.S., in the *Lancet* of November 22nd. The scene is a physiological laboratory. A dog has undergone a terrible experimental operation, —removal of part of the bowels. The operation, though per-

o

formed under anæsthetics, is one which necessarily entails very acute after-sufferings. It is the second night after this opera-tion, and the dog is left in its pain, tied so that it cannot move. But it is not left altogether without a sympathiser. ' During the night another dog, tied up in the same room, slipped his collar, and bit through the cord which secured the subject of the experiment.' At ten o'clock the next morning it was found that ' the dressings were removed, and both dogs had been running about the room.' Let your readers picture to them-selves what happened in the darkness of that awful night. One dog, tied down and unable to stir, is crying in pain. Another —awaiting the same fate—hearing the cries, struggles till it frees itself to go to the sufferer's help. Thinking the cords that bind it may be the cause of its pain, it gnaws them through. Next, the dressings are torn off ; and as this brings no relief, the victim rushes round the room in its agony, with its sym-pathising friend at its side. At last it can run no longer ; and the experimenter, on his arrival, finds it lying on its side. ' The abdomen was tympanitic, and very painful to the touch.' It is a comfort to learn that the dog died at 11.45 a.m., after a dose of atropia given with the object of producing that result. Thus ended the tragedy. The ' subject of the experiment ' was, we are told, a black-and-tan bitch, weighing 16·3 lbs. The ' subject ' of the next experiment—in all likelihood the sympathising friend of the first—' a bitch weighing 16·3 lbs.' The powers of love and sympathy in the hearts of these creatures and their sensitiveness to pain, cannot be *weighed*, and so do not enter into the calculations of the experimenters. All the experiments failed."—Letter in *The Spectator* (Nov. 29th, 1884).

PAIN in Animals as acutely felt as in Human Beings.   Pritchard.

WILLIAM PRITCHARD, M.R.C.S., F.C.S. (the late), Professor of Anatomy at the Royal Veterinary College. (A.V.)

" You must have studied the animal frame very attentively ; have you formed any definite idea as to the comparative sensi-tiveness to pain of different animals, as for instance between a horse and a dog ?—Well, I have performed some thousands of operations on them, and I have never yet been able to detect any difference in sensation between the skin of either one or the other, and the human subject, beyond this, that the cuticle or external covering of the skin is thicker in some animals than in others, and of course the knife has to penetrate deeper to reach the sensitive structure ; but when once it has reached the

sensitive structure I think it is as sensitive in the one animal as the other. And you think that as regards the mere physical sensation of pain it would be equal to that in a human being ?—Yes. I have never seen anything to lead me to think otherwise. Have you any opinion as to what it would be in the case of frogs ?—I think there would be a sensation to a similar extent. That they would be as sensitive as horses ?—Yes. What is your reason for thinking so ?—We find that the irritation of a parasite on the external surface produces as great an irritation in the small animals as it does in the larger ones."
—*Evid. Roy. Com.* (London, 1876), Q. 846-50.

PAIN—Prolonged. Fergusson.

SIR WILLIAM FERGUSSON, Bart., F.R.S. (the late), Sergeant Surgeon to the Queen (born 1808 ; died 1877). (A.V.)

" We have been told that, speaking generally, experiments of this kind are performed with the greatest possible consideration for the animal, and with the greatest indisposition to inflict at least protracted suffering. Do you believe that to be the case ? Gentlemen may fancy that, but I do not think that they fulfil that idea. Indeed, I have reason to imagine that such sufferings, incidental to such operations, are protracted in a very shocking manner. I will give an illustration of an animal being crucified for several days perhaps ; introduced several times into a lecture room for the class to see how the experiment was going on."—*Evid. Roy. Com.* (London, 1876), Q. 1,057.

—— **The same.**—*See also* ABNORMAL CONDITION OF VIVISECTED ANIMALS.

—— The same.—Cases where cannot be Humphry. Alleviated.

SIR G. M. HUMPHRY, M.D., F.R.C.S., F.R.S., Professor of Surgery, Cambridge University. (V.)

" You implied, I think, that pathological experiments were sometimes as painful as physiological experiments ; did I understand you to say that the anæsthetic practice is as applicable to pathology as it is to physiology ?—I think not, because the process may have to be observed during some days. *Mr. Hutton :* Or weeks ?—Yes. or weeks. *Lord Winmarleigh :* You do not think that the pain of pathological experiments can be alleviated in the same manner ?—Not to the same extent."—*Evid. Roy. Com.* (London, 1876), Q. 667-9.

PAIN—Sensitiveness of Animals to. Sanderson.

J. BURDON SANDERSON, M.D., F.R.S., Regius Professor of Medicine, Oxford University. (V.)

" With regard to experiments on inflammation, even the most simple ones cannot be done without the production of a certain amount of pain, because pain is one of the phenomena of inflammation. Does that imply . . . that the experiment cannot be performed under anæsthetics ?—With anæsthesia as regards many other operations perhaps, but still without anæsthesia as regards the process itself. You cannot produce an inflammation in an animal and maintain a state of anæsthesia during the whole of the process. It is quite impossible."—*Evid. Roy. Com.* (London, 1876),Q. 2,298, 9.

—— The same—Any amount justifiable Carpenter. according to some.

W. B. CARPENTER, C.B., M.D. (the late), Registrar of London University (born 1812 ; died 1885). (V.)

" Would you put any limit on the painful character of the experiments to be made for a scientific purpose ? I should certainly justify the infliction of any amount of pain for a sufficient scientific purpose," etc.* (Q. 5,603.)

In answer to Question 5,627, he says :—" . . . I have myself seen in certain instances a perfect callousness to animal suffering before the introduction of anæsthetics. I will not mention names, but I have seen a callousness which very strongly repelled me, and this when important experiments were being performed. But that, I think, does not constitute any adequate reason against the performance of well-considered experiments with a definite object." At Question 5,616, Dr. Carpenter is asked : "I see an experiment narrated in your own work on physiology, as to which I should like to know whether you think it was a really desirable one to make. I find this stated—' The introduction of a little boiling water threw the animal at once into a kind of a dynamic state, which was followed by death in three or four hours ; the mucous membrane of the stomach was found red and swollen,'

---

* It must have been this and similar evidence which inspired Mr. Richard Holt Hutton to write his exceedingly important rider to the Report (signed by himself alone). He sums up his plea for the protection of such domestic animals as dogs and cats in these words ; "Indeed, I may be allowed to say that the measure proposed will not at all satisfy my own conception of the needs of the case, unless it results in putting an end to all experiments involving, not merely torture, but anything at all approaching it ; for where the pursuit of scientific truth and common compassion come into collision it seems to me that the ends of civilisation, no less than of morality, require us to be guided by the latter and higher principle."

etc. . . . It is not one of your own experiments, but one of which you are there narrating the results. Now, do you not think that that might have been argued as one of the most certain inferences from the well-known facts of human experience, and that it was quite an unnecessary experiment to make?"—"That which you have just read is probably taken from a late edition of my book (seventh edition by Mr. Power)." Q. 5,619: "It is published in your book, but not by you?"—"Not by me."*

Further evidence of Dr. Carpenter's is to the following effect :—Q. 5,621 : " . . . Various experiments on glueing animals together—that is to say, removing the skin from two different animals, and binding them closely together, so that a new membrane forms, which is common to both . . . until they grow together in fact. . . . Clearly it must involve the greatest possible misery to the animals so artificially united?" [Professor Huxley remarks that experiments such as these have been made to put Darwin's theory of *pangenesis* to the test.] 5,624: "Do you not think that there may be some danger that a physiologist would be inclined to try experiments (I mean painful experiments) simply with a sort of discovering idea, to find out what will happen, without having any definite notion of producing a result which would bear upon some question affecting life or pain?"—"I am quite sure that that has been the case, and is the case." 5,625 : " And would you not consider that that is a thing open to very great objection?"—"Certainly."—*Evid. Roy. Com.* (London, 1876).

PAIN—What a Vivisector does not consider.   Sibson.

FRANCIS SIBSON, M.D., F.R.S. (the late). (V.)

" Dr. Sibson asked (Q. 4,745): 'I suppose you would not deny that the sufferings involved in raising the temperature of animals till they died would be very severe?' gave it as his belief that but little suffering is caused by raising the temperature, because ' by the time the animal acquires anything like a temperature of 110, 111, or 112, the animal becomes unconscious.' Q. 4,746 : ' The intermediate period is one of great suffering, I suppose ? '—' In the intermediate period the sufferings are not great.' Dr. Sibson goes on to say that freezing animals to death, and starving them to death (Mangili's and Chossat's experiments),would not cause pain."—*Evid. Roy. Com.*(London, 1876).

* It subsequently appeared that Dr. Carpenter's memory was in fault, and that the story had appeared in an earlier edition of his book.

PAIN—Escape from, not a Proper Object.   Huxley.

THOMAS HENRY HUXLEY, M.R.C.S., LL.D., Professor and
    Dean, Science and Art Department, South Kensington.   (V.)

"If we may permit ourselves a larger hope of abatement of
the essential evil of the world than was possible to those who,
in the infancy of exact knowledge, faced the problem of existence more than a score of centuries ago, I deem it an essential
condition of the realisation of that hope that we should cast
aside the notion that the escape from pain and sorrow is the
proper object of life.—*Huxley's* "*Collected Essays*," vol. ix.,
pp. 85-6 (London, 1894).

—— And Pleasure in Animals.   Voltaire.

FRANCOIS M. AROUET de VOLTAIRE, French Author and
    Philosopher (born 1694 ; died 1778).   (A.V.)

"Is it from my speaking that you allow me sense, memory,
and ideas? Well, I am silent; but you see me come home
very melancholy, and with eager anxiety look for a paper, open
the bureau where I remember to have put it, and read it with
apparent joy. You hence infer that I have felt pain and
pleasure, and think I have memory and knowledge. Make the
like reference concerning this dog, which, having lost his
master, searches for him in all the streets with cries of sorrow,
and comes home agitated and restless ; he goes upstairs,
downstairs, runs from room to room, till at length he finds his
beloved master in his closet, and betokens his gladness by his
soft whispers, his gesticulations, his caresses. This dog, so very
superior to man in his affection, is seized by some barbarian
virtuosos, who nail him down to a table, and dissect him while
living, the better to show you the mezeraic veins. All the
same organs of sensation which are in yourselves you perceive
in him. Now, our automatonists (*machinistes*), what say you?
Answer me. Has nature created all the springs of feeling
in this animal, that it may not feel? Has he nerves to be
without pleasure or pain? For shame! Charge not nature
with such weakness or inconsistency."—"*Dictionnaire Philoso-
phique*," *English translation* (London, T. Brown, 1765), pp. 29-30.

—— In Animals.   Ruffer.

MARC ARMAND RUFFER, M.A., M.D., London.   (V.)

That animals are capable of suffering intense pain, amounting to torture, is evidenced by Dr. Ruffer, who tells us of "the

horses which remained in a mangled condition on the battle-field, and which suffered torture for weeks." This is important, because an attempt is often made by physiologists to make us believe that "pain is far less appreciated by animals than by man."—E. BELL, in the "*Contemporary Review*," Dec., 1892.

PAIN in Animals.   "Lancet."

"THE LANCET," London. (V.)

" It is positively sickening to read of a poor bird, clumsily accoutred, cutting its own throat with the sharp steel spur intended for the destruction of its antagonist."—*Lancet*, April 26th, 1884, *on Cockfighting*.

—— The same.   Hart.

ERNEST ABRAHAM HART, Editor the *British Medical Journal*, London. (P.V.)

"A proper field for the merciful energies of those who are humanely desirous of minimising to the utmost the pain now daily and hourly inflicted upon animals for the service and convenience of man would be the prevention of unnecessary pain—which is cruelty—in the operations of the farmyard and the household."—*British Medical Journal*, Nov. 26th, 1892, p. 1192.

—— The same.   Bell.

ERNEST BELL, London. (A.V.)

" Physiologists, by their wholesale condemnation of all cruelties except their own, indicate their real opinion with regard to capacity of suffering in animals, and several have made incautious admissions of the agony caused by their own experiments. Prof. Barrow, an ardent advocate of vivisection, is apparently no disbeliever in animal pain, for he has been president of the Ryde Society for the Protection of Animals. Mantegazza has been president of the Italian Society for the Protection of Animals, and Prof. Schiff, one of the most reck-less of foreign vivisectors, was also a member of the Geneva S.P.C.A.

PAINFUL EXPERIMENTS.—*See* CRUEL.

PASTEUR'S LIMITATIONS.—*See* HYDROPHOBIA.

PATIENTS,—*See also* " HOSPITAL PATIENTS " and " HUMAN BEINGS."

PATIENTS—Experiments on.—The Grafting of Cancercus Tumours.—*See* CANCER GRAFTING.

PITY—The Practice of Vivisection   Macaulay, represses the Emotion of.

JAMES MACAULAY, M.A., M.D., F.R.C.S.Ed., London.   (A.V.)

" It is a law in ethics, that the strength of any motive is increased or diminished according to the habitual exercise of the mental emotion brought into play.   Sympathy for distress and aversion to inflict pain may be naturally strong in the heart of a biologist or physician, but may be gradually overpowered and suppressed by the habitual exercise of other motives, such as zeal for science or ambition of scientific fame.   Every time these passions prevail an increased purchase is gained for their future influence, and the heart is hardened as they encroach on the rightful domain of sympathy and compassion for poor suffering animals.   In other persons, the better feeling of possibly rendering good to men by improvements in medicine represses the immediate emotion of pity; and even humane physicians advocate the most fearful proceedings of vivisection."—" *Vivisection, A Prize Essay* (London, 1881), p. 82.

PODOPHYLLIN—Confusion created   Berdoe. by Experiments with.

EDWARD BERDOE, M.R.C.S., L.R.C.P.Ed., London.   (A.V.)

" This well-known drug has been the subject of many investigations as to its action upon the liver.   Dr. Anstie studied its action on dogs and cats.   Writing of these experiments Dr. Ringer says (p. 385), ' The animals suffered great pain, and soon became exhausted.'   They vomited violently, their intestines were congested, inflamed, and ulcerated by the injection of an alcoholic solution of the drug into the abdomen ; and as the result of these atrociously cruel experiments, Dr. Anstie came to the conclusion that podophyllin was not a cholagogue, that is to say, it did not increase the secretion of bile.   Rohrig performed more experiments, the results of which were opposed to the statements of Anstie, and Professor Rutherford began his long series of vivisections upon dogs for the Edinburgh Committee, endeavouring to reconcile the conflicting results of other experimenters. ' These experiments,' says Dr. Stillé (p. 1124), have led to diametrically opposite results.' "—*The Futility of Experiments with Drugs on Animals*, by Edward Berdoe (London, 1889), pp. 32-3.

POISON OAK *(Rhus Toxicodendron)*—   Berdoe.
Varying Effects of, on Animals
and Human Beings.

EDWARD BERDOE, M.R.C.S., L.R.C.P.Ed., London. (A.V.)

"'The medicinal virtues of this plant are too uncertain to inspire any confidence.'—*(Stillé*, p. 1464.) Dogs have died after being merely exposed to the emanations of this plant, and they are poisoned by its juice, yet herbivorous animals devour its leaves with impunity, and it is recorded that two children, who between them had eaten a pint of the berries, were not killed by them, though they became delirious and convulsed."—*The Futility of Experiments with Drugs on Animals*, by Edward Berdoe (London, 1889), p. 33.

POISON—Detection of.   Tait.

LAWSON TAIT, F.R.C.S., late Professor of Gynæcology, Queen's College, Birmingham. (A.V.)

" I have looked in vain for any record of a research for a method which will detect aconitine with certainty by chemical analysis, as strychnine can be detected, and Dr. Stephenson admitted in evidence that there was no such test. I daresay such a method will be shortly published.

     ❊   ❊   ❊   ❊   ❊

"At present, when need arises, we must go back to the uncertain method of experimenting upon animals. But this is not science, if by that word we are to speak of exact knowledge.

     ❊   ❊   ❊   ❊   ❊

" The general conclusion therefore is, that for such purposes experiments on animals should be entirely prohibited, and that an exhaustive research should at once be undertaken at the expense of the State, upon the spectrum and chemical analysis of all substances which may be used for criminal purposes. There is no known substance of constant character which has resisted the chemist's effort to identify it when it has been properly investigated."—" *Uselessness of Vivisection*," by L. Tait (Birmingham, 1882), pp. 38, 39.

—— The same—Experiments with, on   Watson.
Animals useless.

SIR THOMAS WATSON, Bart., M.D. (the late), Ex-President Royal College of Physicians (born 1792 ; died 1882). (V.)

" But does it follow that because any drug would be

poisonous to a dog it would necessarily be poisonous to
a man ?—No, not at all. On that account I think it was that
you said that you had no great faith in experiments made
of the effects of drugs upon animals ?—No, I should not have
any faith in such experiments.—*Evid. Roy. Com.* (London, 1876),
Q. 57, 58.

POISONS—Experiments with, on   Taylor.
Animals useless.

ALFRED SWAYNE TAYLOR (the late), M.D., F.R.C.P., F.R.S.
(born 1806 ; died 1880). (P.V.)

" Do you think that, speaking of toxicological experiments,
when performed even by men of great names in science, they
are always necessary and really conducive to scientific results ?
—They are not always so. They may have an intention of
working out some problem in their own minds ; but as for
being of general use in science, they certainly are not so ;
a number of experiments, in fact, are uselessly performed.
Would you give us an illustration ?—I would say that was the
case chiefly among the French authorities, and without
perhaps naming individuals, I may say that a very eminent
toxicologist was in the habit of experimenting upon dogs on
a very large scale indeed—and after giving the poisons (nearly
every poison in the list that we know of) to the animals by the
mouth, he cut into the neck to tie the æsophagus (the gullet),
to prevent the animal vomiting ; and of course that must have
caused great pain and suffering, and it also prevented the
efforts of nature to get rid of the poison, and at the same
time it defeated the object which a toxicologist ought to have
in view, because it placed the animal in an unnatural
condition ; for one could not fairly judge from the symptoms
what the effects would be from that particular poison. For
that reason in my work on Toxicology I have not been able
to make any use of the hundreds of these experiments which
this French physician performed ; I have only been able
to make use of those observations that were made on human
beings, where the poison was allowed to act in the
usual way without interference. The application of a ligature
to the gullet was attended with great pain and suffering, and
defeated the very object for which he undertook it. He
wanted to prevent vomiting, and in doing that he altered,
of course, all the circumstances which we should study
in regard to a human being. Others have worked since that
time on dogs, but I believe not in quite so cruel a fashion.

Are those kind of experiments really conducive to scientific conclusions or not ?—I can hardly say that they help us much. the results depend so much on the weight of the animal and the circulation of the blood, and so on ; they allow us simply to say this, ' Such a substance is a poison or not.' The toxicologist has tried an experiment with the poison, of serpents or the cobra poison, and it has just allowed him to say, ' This destroys the life of a small animal,' and that does not help us in medical jurisprudence. In fact, I have never quoted, in any evidence that I have given, the results of experiments upon such animals as frogs or birds."—*Evid. Roy. Com.* (London, 1876), Q. 1,170-72.

POISONS—Experiments with, on   Macaulay.
    Animals useless.

JAMES MACAULAY, M.A., M.D., F.R.C.S.Ed., London. (A.V.)

" The discovery of antidotes to poisons is the most plausible ground on which the danger of delay in research can be pleaded. So far as this country is concerned, and in the experience of any general practitioner, ninety-nine in every hundred cases of poisoning, and even a larger proportion, are from substances with which we are perfectly familiar, and the antidotes to which are well known. Our practice in all these cases is intelligently guided by facts of physiology and of chemistry, confirmed by general experience. In very few cases indeed are *specific* antidotes known for poisons, and if any are proposed, their efficiency must be proved in actual practice."—" *Vivisection,*" *A Prize Essay* (London, 1881), pp. 56-7.

—— The same—Rabbits eat Belladonna   Rolleston.
    with impunity.

GEORGE ROLLESTON (the late), M.D., Professor of Anatomy at Oxford (born 1829 ; died 1890). (P.V.)

" A rabbit will eat as much belladonna as would poison a large number of men, and yet it will not act upon the rabbit in the least."—*Evid. Roy. Com.* (London, 1876), Q. 1,280.

PUBLIC PLACE.—See Act, etc.

PRUSSIC ACID *(Hydrocyanic Acid)*—Confusing   Berdoe.
    Results of Experiments with.

EDWARD BERDOE, M.R.C.S., L.R.C.P.Ed., London. (A.V.)

" This, as everybody knows, is one of the most deadly

poisons to human beings, yet on horses and hyænas it has little or no effect. The elephant, however, is destroyed by a relatively small dose.

"Claude Bernard and others said that after poisoning by prussic acid the venous blood of the animals experimented upon was of a *bright arterial hue* at the *post mortem.*—(*Wood*, p. 182.)

"Boëhm and Knil (*Archiv für Exper. Pathol. und Therap. Bd.* ii., p. 137) experimented on cats with this poison and obtained certain results.

"Rossbach and others found that it lowered the frequency of the pulse.

"Wahl found that it increased it.

"Bischoff and other German investigators say that they found nothing but *dark venous blood* either in man or animals so poisoned.—(*Wood*, p. 182.)

"Preyer performed the same kind of experiments on rabbits and obtained quite different results.

"Boëhm and Preyer contradict each other as to the action of this drug on the respiration.

"Kölliker and Stannius are at variance as to its local effects on the nerves.—(*Wood*, p. 187.)

"Some of these experiments were most severe, such as opening the chests of rabbits, and exposing the heart, and then administering the poison."

—*The Futility of Experiments with Drugs on Animals*, by Edward Berdoe (London, 1889), pp. 33-4.

QUININE—Confusing Effects of Experiments with.   Berdoe.

EDWARD BERDOE, M.R.C.S., L.R.C.P.Ed., London. (A.V.)

"Physiologists are not agreed as to the therapeutic action of quinine.

"Professor Binz poisoned a cat with quinine and afterwards examined its blood. He found the white corpuscles much less abundant than those in the blood of an unpoisoned cat.— (*Virchow's Archiv*, Bd. xlvi., p. 137.)

"Schwalbe and Geltowski performed similar experiments, and could detect no difference in the blood before and after poisoning by quinine.—(*Pfluger's Archiv*, Bd. i., p. 203.)

"Binz experimented with quinine on ten dogs and rabbits, and found that it killed the microscopic entities which cause septic diseases.

" Professor Wood says these experiments indicate very clearly that it does nothing of the sort.—(*Wood*, p. 73.)

" It has been maintained by many physicians, and apparently confirmed by experiments on animals, that quinine is ' dangerous and even criminal in any diseases of pregnant women.' —Dr. Jos. J. West (*Savannah Journal of Medicine*, vol. i., p. 19.)

" To test this question, Professor Chiara, of Milan, experimented ' *in his public service* ' with quinine ' on eight women, all in the eighth month of pregnancy.—(*L'Union Médicale*, Nov. 20th, 1873.) Happily no untoward results followed." —*The Futility of Experiments with Drugs on Animals*, by Edward Berdoe (London, 1889), p. 34.

REID, SUFFERINGS OF DR. JOHN. Wilson.

GEORGE WILSON, M.D., F.R.S. (the late), of Edinburgh. (P.V.)

" The month of August was spent like that of July, only with every agony aggravated. . . . He referred pointedly to the seat of his sufferings (from cancer of the tongue) being the same nerves on which he had made so many experiments, and added, ' This is a judgment on me for the sufferings which I inflicted on animals.' To this he recurred at a later period." (p. 237.)

" He went on to add, repeating the statement more than once, that it might seem foolish, but he could not divest his mind of the feeling that there was a special providence in the way in which he had been afflicted. He had devoted peculiar attention to the functions of certain nerves, and had inflicted suffering on many dumb creatures, that he might discover the office of those nerves, and he could not but regard the cancer which had preyed upon them, in his own body, as a heaven-sent, significant message from God, whom otherwise he might have utterly forgotten." (p. 250.)

" —— who would have ventured to foretell—and who is not startled by learning—that Dr. Reid is doomed to die by a disease which repeats upon his own body, not in one but in many ways, the pains and the perils which he had imposed upon the lower animals ? It certainly was remarkable, and many of his medical brethren felt it to be so." (p. 252.)— *From the " Life of Dr. John Reid,"* by *George Wilson, M.D.* (Edinburgh and London, 1852.)

REMORSE (REID'S) FOR HIS OWN VIVISECTIONS.—*See* REID.

REPETITION OF EXPERIMENTS.   Béclard.

JULES BÉCLARD, M.D., Paris, 1842 ; late Professor of Physiology
Med. Faculty, Paris. (V.)

" Bichat has made, in this respect, an experiment on living
animals, which all physiologists have since repeated. A tube
with a turn-cock is introduced and fixed in the trachea of a
dog, and an artery is subsequently opened in the animal. At
first the respiration is allowed free action ; then the turn-cock
is shut, respiration is thereby suspended, and with it the
entrance of the air into the lungs. The blood which issued
from the wound in the artery was first red ; it becomes analogous
to venous blood. When the turn-cock is again opened, the
blood once more takes a bright hue."—*Béclard's Traité Elé-
mentire de Physiologie* " (Paris, 1880), p. 336.

—— The same.   Haughton.

THE REV. SAMUEL HAUGHTON, M.D., Proctor, late Medical
Registrar School of Physic, Univ. of Dublin ; a witness before the
Royal Commission, 1875. (A.V.)

" I believe that a large proportion of the experiments now
performed upon animals in England, Scotland and Ireland,
are unnecessary and clumsy repetitions of well-known results.
Young physiologists in England learn German and read experiments in German journals, and repeat them in this
country."—*Evid. Roy. Com.* (London, 1876), Q. 1,874.

-—— The same.   Cobbe.

FRANCES POWER COBBE, Authoress, Hengwrt, Dolgelly. (A.V.)

" Mr. Cartwright said that ' a large amount of benefit is
acquired by the medical profession from these experiments, and
it is a noteworthy fact that there is *never any need to renew an
experiment when once made.*'
" The following is some of the evidence which the Royal
Commission received on this subject.
" Professor Humphry said (635), ' Experiments have to be
repeated and confirmed many times before a fact is really
established ' ; and (740) agreed with Dr. Ray Lankester that
· the number of experiments must increase very rapidly if
the progress of science is to be kept up.' Dr. Rutherford told
the Commission (2,993), ' Last year for purposes of research I
think I used about 40 dogs.' He has since, in other series of
exactly similar experiments, ' used ' 62. Dr. Lauder Brunton

told the Commission (5,721) he had used ninety cats in one series of experiments, and (5,747) that he had 'used a much larger number for investigating the subject of cholera than 90.' Dr. Crichton Browne said (3,164) that 'forty-six animals' were sacrificed in trying if chloral was antagonistic to picrotoxine—and (3,178) that twenty-nine animals were used in Dr. Ferrier's series. These are the small and modest figures of English vivisection, as admitted before the Royal Commission."*—*Comments on the Debate in the House of Commons, April 4th, 1883, by Frances Power Cobbe* (London, 1883), pp. 9, 10.

REPETITION OF EXPERIMENTS   Sharpey.
Unjustifiable.

WILLIAM SHARPEY (the late), M.D., LL.D., F.R.S., formerly Professor of Physiology in University College, London (born 1802 ; died 1881). (V.)

"When Monsieur Majendie had proved the distinction between the motor and sensory nerves more completely than Sir Charles Bell had proved them, there was no need of any further proof?—No. Therefore any further experiments for that purpose would be a purposeless infliction of pain?—Quite so. . . . Once such facts are fully established, I do not think it justifiable to repeat experiments causing pain to animals ; such experiments as those of Majendie on the nerves, for example, ought not to be repeated when the fact has been once fairly established."—*Evid. Roy. Com.* (London, 1876), Q. 404-5.

RESECTION OF LUNG.   Tait.

LAWSON TAIT, F.R.C.S., LL.D., late Professor of Gynæcology, Queen's College, Birmingham. (A.V.)

"I cannot imagine that any man in his senses would attempt to remove a human lung with a tumour in it. It would not be resection of parts of four ribs which would permit the removal of a tumour sufficiently large to admit of accurate diagnosis ; and I cannot observe, in the literature just at the

---

* I say nothing of the myriads of victims of foreign recklessness, as when Majendie, according to Flourens, sacrificed 4,000 dogs to prove one hypothesis true, and another 4,000 to prove it false, and when Orfila poisoned 6,000 dogs in the course of his researches in toxicology. M. Blatin, quoting the Viennese *Lumière*, says that "it is calculated that the number of animals carried off at Vienna by physiology in 1850, 1851, and 1852, reached 56,000—to wit, dogs, 26,000 ; cats and rabbits, 25,000 ; horses and asses, 5,000. Dr. de Cyon has just told us (*Contemporary Review*, April, 1883, p. 505) that he has performed " an incalculable number of vivisections."—*F. P. C.*

moment accessible, that any other kinds of tumours occur in the lung, save those of hydatid origin, and those of a cancerous nature. If the tumour were hydatid the removal of the lung would be unnecessary. If the tumour proved to be an aneurism the disaster would be awful. . . . The facility with which Dr. Biondi has removed lungs, and parts of lungs, from dogs, guinea-pigs, cats, fowls, pigeons, and sheep, and the absence of mortality from such operations, is likely to be a snare rather than a help. It does not need saying, that the removal of a healthy lung, collapsed by the introduction of air into the pleura, would be a very easy matter, and very different from the removal of a diseased and adherent organ. There would be as much difference as there is between normal ovariotomy and removal of a pyosalpinx. It is perfectly clear that these animals, with their deep and narrow chests, differ very much from us with our wide and shallow cavities, in their power of enduring the accident of acute pneumothorax; certainly they would differ from us immensely in the facility with which pneumonotomy may be performed. Their chests are built for the endurance of the special efforts of great speed, and we have lost those physical characters; and I venture to say that, if acute pneumothorax were suddenly inflicted upon sixty-three healthy adult human beings, death would be the immediate result in the great majority of the experiments."—*Letter in the "British Medical Journal*," June 20th, 1884.

RESPIRATION, Fallacies of Experiments on the. Barclay.

JOHN BARCLAY, M.D. (the late), Edinburgh (born 1758; died 1826). (P.V.)

"In making experiments on live animals, even when the species of respiration is the same as our own, anatomists must often witness phenomena that can be phenomena only of rare occurrence. After considering that the actions of the diaphragm, in ordinary cases are different from its actions in sneezing and coughing, these again different from its actions in laughing and hiccup; after considering that our breathing is varied by heat and cold, by pleasure and pain, by every strong mental emotion, by the different states of health and disease, by different attitudes and different exertions,—we can hardly suppose that an animal under the influence of horror, placed in a forced and unnatural attitude; its viscera exposed to the stimulus of air; its blood flowing out; many of its muscles divided by the knife; and its nervous system driven to violent desultory action from excruciating pain, would exhibit the phenomena of ordinary respiration. In that situation its muscles must produce many effects, not only of violent but irregular action ; and not only the muscles usually employed in performing the function, but also the muscles that occasionally are required to act as auxiliaries. If different anatomists, after seeing different species of animals or different individuals of the same species respiring under different experiments of torture, were each to conclude that the phenomena produced in these cases were analogous to those of ordinary respiration, their differences of opinion as to the motions of ordinary respiration would be immense."—*On the Muscular Motions*, p. 298.

RESTRICTION OF VIVISECTION A FAILURE.

Cobbe.

FRANCES POWER COBBE, Authoress, Hengwrt, Dolgelly. (A.V.)

" To those who have taken part in the vivisection con-troversy since it began in England in 1874, there is no need to address any argument concerning the right policy to be adopted by the opponents of the practice. They know, and no doubt the vivisectors know equally well, that it is a case of ' all or nothing.' The cruel and misleading method of research must either continue to be legalised, and used *as a method*,— with or without a few formalities, possibly harassing to the physiologists, but of little or no practical use to the victims,— or it must be forbidden *as a method*, and Mr. Lawson Tait's aspiration be fulfilled and the practice stopped in the interests of science, so that the energy and skill of investigators may be turned into better and safer channels.

　　※　　　　※　　　　※　　　　※　　　　※

" No restrictive Act of Parliament which human ingenuity may devise can afford efficient protection to animals delivered over to a vivisector. The advocates of restriction fondly imagine that they *can* devise such provisions ; but with all respect for them, we unhesitatingly assert that no one who understands the *purposes and methods of vivisectional research* can believe that such provisions are possible.

　　※　　　　※　　　　※　　　　※　　　　※

" Again, the advocates of restriction fall back on the old fallacy of anæsthetics, and vaguely conceive they could pass a measure forbidding all experiments except on animals under complete anæsthesia. But even a superficial acquaintance with the works of vivisectors shows us that they would be

P

stopped at every turn could such a condition of experiments be really secured. That it could *not* be secured by any conceivable precautions, is almost equally clear.

∗   ∗   ∗   ∗   ∗

" The incentive to vivisection is, unquestionably, in the vast majority of cases, the honour and distinction obtained among the confraternity by successful researches respecting large or small points in physiology—such distinctions culminating in the statue recently erected in Paris to Claud Bernard.

∗   ∗   ∗   ∗   ∗

" The results of vivisection being, according to our unanimous contention, worse than *nil*—misleading and injurious to science —we shall best befriend science itself by closing up that false path altogether and not making a stile to enable travellers to walk there. In pretending merely to restrict it we are practically admitting our opponents' assertion of its utility; and if we do this, we involve ourselves in inextricable difficulties to determine next the point where a little pain,—or a greater pain,—to one animal or to a thousand animals,—ought to be sanctioned to obtain benefit for mankind, and how great or direct that benefit ought to be, and how far it must be likely of attainment. We fight the battle, in short, thenceforth on our enemy's ground ; and must infallibly be pushed back and back, till all the excesses of scientific cruelty be justified ; just as they were by the different witnesses before the Royal Commission.

" Every imaginable law sanctioning in any measure vivisection is not only fallacious as regards the protection of animals, but *demoralizing to the men* who pursue the practice, and injurious to the community which, at one and the same moment, institutes Bands of Mercy, and treats domestic creatures as pets, servants, and playmates, and then is called on to authorize men to dissect them alive as mere parcels of bone and tissue. Either vivisection ought to be wholly scouted and forbidden, or the whole movement on behalf of kindness to animals, which has been the glory of England since the days of Erskine and Martin, ought to be abandoned, and the hypocrisy renounced of caressing a dog to-day and consenting to his vivisection—restricted or unrestricted—to-morrow."—*Extract from " The Fallacy of Restriction applied to Vivisection,"* by Frances Power Cobbe (London, Victoria Street Society, 1886.)

RESTRICTION OF VIVISECTION   Thornhill.
A FAILURE.

MARK THORNHILL, Esq., late Judge of Sakarunpore, Dover. (A.V.)

" If we advocate the total prohibition of vivisection, we can base our advocacy on grounds of the highest morality, we can appeal to the noblest, the purest, the most unselfish feelings of our nature, and experience has proved that, in modern times, and among our own people, such appeals are seldom made in vain. But if we advocate merely the restriction of vivisection, we can hardly appeal to the feelings at all. We certainly cannot make any very effective appeal; nor, that I see, can we base our advocacy on very lofty morality; for the fact that we desire merely to restrict vivisection implies that, to a certain extent, we approve of vivisection. Also that, to a certain extent, we acknowledge the utility of vivisection—for the utility of vivisection is admitted to be its sole justification."— "*Restriction or Prohibition*," by Mark Thornhill (London, Victoria Street Society), p. 10.

RESTRICTION OF VIVISECTION A FAILURE.

White.

MRS. RICHARD P. WHITE, Humanitarian Leader, Philadelphia, U.S.A. (A.V.)

" We feel that the ground which our Society has hitherto held of restricting cruel experimentation upon animals, yet allowing it to a certain extent, is one which we cannot take any longer. We cannot conscientiously ask for the granting of a license to vivisectors, thus legalizing, to some extent, the torture of animals. We say that it is all wrong; that it is against the laws of God to torture a sentient being without its consent, and we should use all our powers in protesting against it, instead of asking that it be legalized. Moreover, we put ourselves in a false and unfortunate position by taking this ground. Our opponents can say to us with truth: 'You acknowledge that you are in favour of vivisection to a certain extent;' and when we would indignantly disclaim such a supposition, they can reply, 'Why, of course you do; you ask for a license for vivisectors, and you say that your society is for the restriction of vivisection; then you acknowledge that it is right to a certain extent, or you would not say the restriction, but the cessation, of vivisection in your title and in your charter. Now, then, you think it allowable to a certain extent, and we think it allowable to a greater extent; and we have just as much reason to claim that we are in the right as you have.' Allowing, then, that the position which the Society has hitherto taken is a false one, there remain only two grounds for us to adopt—one, the total abolition of all experiments, the other, the total abolition of all painful experiments. . . . Let us take the upright and conscientious ground of refusing all compromise with sin and evil, and, maintaining our position unflinchingly, leave the rest to God." (A resolution adopting total prohibition as the object of the Society was adopted on the 30th December, 1887).—*Extract from Speech of Mrs. White, " Zoophilist,"* January, 1888.

RESULTS—Absence of Good.   Macaulay.

JAMES MACAULAY, M.A., M.D., F.R.C.S.Ed., London.   (A.V.)

" If vivisection were really the luminous and fruitful method of research which its advocates represent it to be, physiology must ere now have been the most advanced of the sciences, and none of the mysteries of animal life would remain obscure. For the last fifty years, on the Continent, many men of high rank in science, learned and gifted, with well appointed laboratories and an unlimited supply of subjects for experiment—encouraged and applauded by the profession, and with no check or restraint from law or public opinion—have zealously cultivated this field of inquiry.   In recent years many physiologists and biologists in England and America have entered into rivalry with those of France, Germany, and Italy.   The experiments during the past half-century may be reckoned by tens of thousands, some say even hundreds of thousands.   Surely we may expect to have obtained abundant fruits from all this expenditure of labour and skill, of time and of life !   Surely we may ask, what are the results of this long and unfettered investigation ? . . . If unquestioned and important results could be shown, the protests against vivisection from the medical profession would be few.   But vivisection has been tried and found wanting."— *Vivisection, A Prize Essay* (London, 1881), p. 70.

RETURNS of Vivisectors are Misleading.   Williams.

WILLIAM WILLIAMS, Principal of the New Veterinary College at Edinburgh ; a witness before the Royal Commission, 1875. (V.)

(Q. 6,084) : " I have here before me the return which you made to the inquiries. . . .   One of the questions is, ' State what animals (including frogs) are used either for original research or class demonstration,' . . .   the reply to which is ' Frogs only ' ? " Mr. Williams answers : " Yes ; that is written by Dr. Young.   I never thought of the horse at the time, the thing really escaped my memory." (6,085) : " In signing that you forgot it ?—Yes." (6,086) : " And you, I suppose, also forgot what had happened when you sent the next answer, in which it is said that the animals are always rendered unconscious ?— Yes."—*Evid. Roy. Com.* (London, 1876).

RETURNS of Vivisectors are Misleading. Sanderson.

JOHN BURDON SANDERSON, M.D., F.R.S., Regius Professor of Medicine, Oxford University. (V.)

" I am able to form a very correct opinion as to the number of people who are actually engaged in this country in physiological investigation. About the time that Dr. Sharpey was giving evidence here, we went through the number together, and at that time we calculated that in England and Scotland there were about thirteen persons now engaged, more or less, in physiological investigations in this country. I think I may make it up, by taking a great deal of pains, to fifteen or sixteen." He then names fifteen, and is asked by Mr. Hutton (2,608) : " Dr. Wickham Legg you have not mentioned ? " " I ought to have put him in ; I forgot him. . . ." Another commissioner (Lord Winmarleigh) adds (2,160) : " As you are giving the whole list, had you not better put in your own name, too? ' " Yes."—*Evid. Roy. Com.* (London, 1876).

RETURNS OF LICENSES AND CERTIFICATES AND EXPERIMENTS MADE. Government Inspectors.

ENGLAND AND SCOTLAND.

LICENSES AND CERTIFICATES.

Year referred to.	Persons Licensed.	No. of Licensees who Experimented.	Certificates Granted.					
			A1	B2	C3	D4	E5	F6
1876	23	no return.	1	—	13	—		—
1877	20	,,	7	13	11	2	7	
1878	45	27	11	14	18	3	6	
1879	36	26	9	6	16	2	—	
1880	33	26	3	8	17	1	1	
1881	38	24	6	8	18	—	1	
1882	42	26	13	12	21	—	2	
1883	44	32	4	23	17	—	2	
1884	49	34	11	16	23	—	4	
1885	53	44	20	20	21	—	10	
1886	66	54	28	25	21	—	16	
1887	82	64	41	22	22	—	17	
1888	75	55	38	21	19	—	—	
1889	87	66	43	34	15	—	18	4
1890	110	77	60	46	14	—	24	3
1891	152	109	98	64	31	2	34	6
1892	180	125	92	75	24	1	39	4
1893	184	135	120	102	32	2	59	3

1-6 See notes on next page.

RETURNS OF LICENSES AND CERTIFICATES AND EXPERIMENTS MADE.

Government Inspectors.

ENGLAND AND SCOTLAND.

EXPERIMENTS MADE.

Year referred to.	Under Licenses alone.	Under Certificates.						Inspector's Total.	T'tа by Simple Addition.	No. o Acmittedly painful Experiments.
		A1	B2	C3	D4	E5	F6			
1876	no return	—	—	—	—	—		—	—	—
1877	,,	—	—	—	—	—		—	—	—
1878	317	87	30	47	—	ircl. in col. 1		481	481	40
1879	126	35	24	61	—	—		270	246	25
1880	174	79	35	60	42*	0		311	348	110†
1881	59	29	92	90	—	1		270	271	122†
1882	118	219	40	29	—	incl. in col. 2		406	406	20 to 30†
1883	256	55	122	—	—	102		535	535	22 or 23†
1884	140	145	76	78	—	2		441	441	18†
1885	210	382	128	82	—	9‡		800	802	35 or 40†
1886	297	458	213	70	—	57		1035	1095§	40†
1887	357	582	162	46	—	73		1220	1220	71
1888	239	498	195	82	—	25	30	1069	1069	8
1889	428	644	170	75	—	18	19	1417	1417	88†
1890	872	796	255	57	—	112	10	2102	2102	316
1891	875	1363	210	211	—	94	8	2661	2661	no return.
1892	1046	2239	303	125	—	224	18	3960	3960	,,
1893	1061	2183	317	140	—	341	4	4046	4046	,,

1 Special for experiments without anæsthetics.

2 Dispensing with the obligation to kill the animal before recovering from anæsthesia.

3 Certificates permitting experiments in illustration to lectures (use of anæsthetics obligatory).

4 For the further advancement of knowledge by testing previous di coveries.

5 Permitting experiments on cats or dogs, without anæsthetics.

6 Permitting experiments on horses, mules or asses.

* These 42 are stated to be included in the number of experiments performed under licenses, and hence are not included in either total.

† The report of these cases is accompanied with a notification that the pain inflicted was in some slight only.

‡ These are stated to be included in col. 2, and are not therefore included in either total.

§ In a second return for 1886, the simple addition total was adopted by the Inspector.

RETURNS OF LICENSES AND CERTIFICATES AND EXPERIMENTS MADE.

Government Inspectors.

IRELAND.

Year.	Persons Licensed.	No. of Licensees who Experimented.	Certificates Granted.				
			A1	B2	C3	D4	E5
1876	—	—	—	—	—	—	—
1877	8	—	—	—	3	--	—
1878	10	5	—	—	20	--	--
1879	8	1	1	—	—	--	--
1880	7	6	—	—	10	—	—
1881	6	4	—	—	13	--	—
1882	5	--	—	—	—	—	—
1883	4	4	1	—	—	—	--
1884	4	2	—	—	—	—	--
1885	3	1	—	—	—	—	—
1886	3	3	—	—	—	—	—
1887	4	3	—	—	—	—	—
1888	4	1	—	—	—	—	--
1889	4	3	—	—	1	—	--
1890	5	3	—	—	—	--	—
1891	5	3	—	2	—	--	2
1892	3	2	—	2	—	—	1
1893	4	2	—	—	—	--	—

1-5 See notes on previous page.

RETURNS, OFFICIAL, The Value of.

Coleridge.

LORD COLERIDGE, Q.C., London. (A.V.)

The Hon. B. (now Lord) Coleridge, speaking at the Annual Meeting of the Victoria Street Society on the 12th June, 1885, criticised the official returns in the following terms :—

" Now, ladies and gentlemen, I propose to direct your attention to one brief point. You may all of you know that whenever we go about and ask persons to join our Society, we are always met by the argument that all cruelty is avoided by the Cruelty to Animals Act of 1876, and they point with triumphant exultation to the report of the Inspector for the year to prove the truth of their conclusions. Now, ladies and gentlemen, with great brevity I will go through the reports, year by year, and I think I shall satisfy you, and if I satisfy you, I hope you will satisfy all your questioners, that these reports are utterly misleading, and that they do not give anything like a true history of the state of affairs which is going on around us.

In the year 1878, Mr. Busk told us that ' in sixteen cases alone, as far as he was able to judge,—and those were confined to two sets of experiments,—in sixteen cases alone was there reason to believe any considerable amount or suffering was directly inflicted.' Now, in that very year, from January to June, Dr. Gaskell, of Cambridge, who did not appear upon that report as a licensee, and therefore had no right at law to vivisect at all, experimented on dogs, using curare, for the purpose of making experiments on the vaso-motor nerves. You will see of how much value the report of that year was ! In the year 1879 the Inspector told us that the number of experiments in which any material suffering was caused was about twenty-five, and of those fifteen were diseases caused by inoculation. In that year one professor, and one professor alone, experimented upon more animals by inoculation than the whole of the number which is here talked of by Inspector Busk, and he experimented upon them with regard to discoveries about anthrax, which Professor Tyndall has told us causes the very greatest suffering. Professor Tyndall tells us that ' it is a loathsome disease ; that the sufferings of animals dying from it are obviously very great, and that an account of the symptoms which precede death would, by no means, be pleasant reading.' I think with regard to the year 1879 this report seems to be equally misleading. In the year 1880 we are told that there were seventy-nine experiments in all, of which ' sixty-nine consisted in simple inoculation (no more painful than ordinary vaccination), which in thirty-eight cases was followed by no ill effect whatever ' ; but that in about thirty instances ' disease appears to have ensued which, during the brief period the animals survived, may have caused slight suffering.' In that year, Professor Greenfield published an account of his operations concerning anthrax, and the remarks of Professor Tyndall with regard to the suffering which they cause are equally applicable to it. In that year there were the terrible sufferings caused by the experiments with regard to the pathology of the spleen, with which we are all familiar ! In the year 1882, we are told that the amount of direct pain inflicted was altogether trifling ; and was limited to ' between twenty and thirty animals, mostly frogs.' In that year, Dr. Watson Cheyne, during the months of August, September, October, and November, performed a series of experiments by putting setons with calf lymph and various poisons into the eyes of rabbits and guinea-pigs. During that year, Dr. Ringer, who held no license, and had no legal qualifications for performing a single experiment, experimented on more than

seventy frogs. Of what value is the report of Mr. Busk of that
year ? In the year 1883, we are told by Mr. Busk that ' the
amount of direct or indirect suffering,' was ' wholly insignificant, and limited to about fourteen or fifteen animals.' In that
year, Drs. Ringer and Murrell, without a license and with no
legal qualifications, experimented with nitrite of sodium and
with various other chemicals upon cats and frogs ; and they
went further, and with true logical consistency applied their
experiments to men and to women at one of the hospitals. Now,
coming down to the last year, 1884, we are told that ' the
amount of direct or indirect suffering ' was ' wholly insignificant.' Mr. Busk reports five experiments only of immersion
of fish in distilled water ' which proved fatal to about thirty
minnows and sticklebacks.' Dr. Ringer alone tells us that he
experimented on 687 fish, and if Dr. Ringer is right, of what
value are the reports of Mr. Busk ? It is the system which is
at fault. What would the working men of this country say if
the inspection of factories and of mines rested upon the statements of the owners of the factories and of the mines ? What
would result to our education if the inspection of our national
schools rested entirely upon the statements of the teachers
themselves of the wonderful performances which were taking
place under their eyes ? Why, gentlemen, we should know at
once that all such reports, founded on such statements, were
wholly illusory."—*Speech at Annual Meeting of the Victoria Street
Society*, June 12th, 1885.

RETURNS, VALUE OF THE OFFICIAL. Clarke.

JOHN H. CLARKE, M.D., Physician to the Homœopathic Hospital,
London. (A.V.)

" Mr. Collier seems to be under the impression that the
Official Report on Vivisection is a trustworthy document.
That this is not the case most doctors and all medical students
well know. In the year 1882, during which the Report tells us
' the amount of direct pain or suffering inflicted in the prosecution of physiological, pathological, and therapeutical researches through the year was altogether trifling, and limited
to between twenty and thirty animals, mostly frogs,' Mr.
Watson Cheyne conducted his tubercle research. He experimented on sixty-eight animals—thirty-seven rabbits, twenty-
five guinea-pigs, one cat, and five mice. Of the thirty-seven
rabbits, twenty-eight had tubercular matter, vaccine virus, bits
of thread, and other substances introduced into their eyes—
six of them into both eyes, a different substance into each for

comparison : of the guinea-pigs, twelve had similar substances, and, in some instances, pieces of cork introduced into the abdominal cavity ; the cat had something injected into its abdominal cavity, and the mice had diseased matter placed into cuts made in the skin. No anæsthetics were used. The account of these experiments is to be found in the *Practitioner* for April, 1883, and any one who wishes to know what the Report is worth should compare the sickening details with the words of the Inspector. The latter draws his information from the experimenters themselves. This is merely a single instance in which it is possible from published statements to check the Report."— *Letter to "Spectator,"* May 3rd, 1884.

RETURNS—Value of the Official. Clarke.

JOHN H. CLARKE, M.D., Physician to the Homœopathic Hospital, London. (A.V.)

" Like all British defenders of vivisection, he (' Philan-thropos ') points with glee to the Returns furnished by Mr. Busk. We have again and again proved that these returns are not to be trusted, and will only add here one word concerning them. In his last report (1883), Mr. Busk states, referring to the experiments we have quoted above from the *Practitioner*, and many others there recorded as bad or worse :—

" 'The only operative proceeding consisting in simple inoculation with a morbid virus by hypodermic injection, would be scarcely felt. The only suffering in these cases would arise from the after consequences of the inoculation, etc., in the production of disease. . . . The suffering, if any, would be of very brief duration, as the animal would either die or be at once killed. As a matter of fact, I have been assured by the experimenters that in this class no appreciable pain was manifested.'

" When our readers recollect the months of suffering endured by the animals in the tubercle research which we have noticed above, and compare it with Mr. Busk's ' brief ' suffering, ' if any,' they will be able to appreciate at once his reliableness in statements of plain matters of fact, such as time, and in pronouncing an opinion on the amount of pain endured by the animals. And, again, when it is remembered that a large number of these injections of variously horrible substances, which Mr. Busk calls hypodermic (*i.e.* under the skin), were not hypodermic at all, but were made into the eyes of the animals, or into the abdominal cavity, it will be seen how naturally ' Philanthropos ' will appeal to Mr. Busk when he is in want of ' facts ' to suit the purposes of his arguments." " *Physiological Cruelty* : " *A Reply to* " *Philanthropos* " (London, 1883), pp. 44, 5.

RIGHTS OF ANIMALS.   Bell.

ERNEST BELL, London. (A.V.)

" That animals have rights is practically admitted by all civilised nations which have societies for the prevention of cruelty, and by all individuals who admit that vivisection should be in any way restricted. If any one argues that the protection afforded animals is an act of clemency, not an admission of their rights, he places himself in an absurd position, for if an animal has no rights, then a man is at liberty to do with it what he pleases, and in obstructing him one is infringing his right. Unless, therefore, we are prepared to allow unlimited cruelty, we are in consistency bound to admit that animals have certain rights, if men have, which rights are regulated as in the case of men, not by the animals-power of reciprocating them, but by their power of enjoying them, and are limited by the necessity of not infringing the similar rights of others."

—— The same.   Salt.

H. S. SALT, Hon. Secretary Humanitarian League, London. (A.V.)

" If ' rights ' exist at all—and both feeling and usage indubitably prove that they do exist—they cannot be consistently awarded to men and denied to animals, since the same sense of justice and compassion applies in both cases. ' Pain is pain,' says an honest old writer (Humphry Primatt, D.D.), ' whether it be inflicted on man or on beast ; and the creature that suffers it, whether man or beast, being sensible of the misery of it while it lasts, suffers evil ; and the sufferance of evil, unmeritedly, unprovokedly, where no offence has been given, and no good can possibly be answered by it, but merely to exhibit power or gratify malice, is cruelty and injustice in him that occasions it."—*Animals' Rights* (London, 1892), p. 24.

—— The same.—*See also* ANIMALS' RIGHTS.

SALIVA, HUMAN—Fatal Effects of.   Sternberg.

GEORGE M. STERNBERG, M.D., Surgeon and Major, U.S.A. (V.)

" I have demonstrated by repeated experiments that my

saliva in doses of 1·25 c.c. to 1·75 c.c. injected into subcutaneous connective tissue of a rabbit, *infallibly produces death*,
usually within forty-eight hours. . . . The saliva of four
students, residents of Baltimore, gave negative results; eleven
rabbits injected with the saliva of six individuals in Philadelphia
gave eight deaths and three negative results; but in the fatal
cases a less degree of virulence was shown in six cases by a
more prolonged period between the date of injection and the
date of death."—*American Journal of Medical Sciences*, July,
1882, pp. 71, etc.

SALIVA, HUMAN—*See also* INOCULATIONS.

—— HEALTHY, causes Death. Vulpian.

A. VULPIAN, M.D. (the late), Professor of Comparative and
Experimental Pathology, Medical Faculty of Paris. (V.)

" M. Vulpian injected under the skin of rabbits saliva
collected at the very moment of the experiment, from perfectly
healthy individuals, and this injection killed the rabbit so
inoculated in forty-eight hours. The blood of these rabbits
was found to be filled with microscopic organisms; among
which was a special organism discovered by M. Pasteur in the
course of his experiments with inoculation of the saliva
of a child who had died of rabies. One drop of this blood,
diluted in ten grammes of distilled water, and injected under
the skin of other rabbits, also brought on the death of these
animals; the blood of which was similarly filled with
microscopic organisms."—*British Medical Journal*, April 9th,
1881, p. 571.

SARSAPARILLA—Fruitlessness of Berdoe.
Experiments with.

EDWARD BERDOE, M.R.C.S., L.R.C.P.Ed., London. (A.V.)

" Doctors are not agreed as to the question of the efficacy
of this drug, and though some surgeons still hold by it, the
physiologists are sceptical as to its uses.
" Palotta experimented with it, and found its alkaloid
produce gastric disturbance, vomiting and slowing of the pulse.
" Bœcker found it to be devoid of physiological activity and
therapeutic power.—(*Bartholow's Materia Medica*, p. 225.)"
— *The Futility of Experiments with Drugs on Animals*, by
Edward Berdoe (London, 1889), p. 35.

SCARLATINA—Inutility of Discovery of Microbe of.　　　Dowdeswell.

GEORGE FRANCIS DOWDESWELL, M.A., F.R.S., etc. (the late). (V.)

"Quite recently, too, it has been asserted, in two different investigations, that, in scarlatina, a microbe is the *materies morbi;* and yet, as if to demonstrate the practical inutility of these investigations, we are, immediately upon the statement, visited by as severe and *unmanageable* an outbreak of this disease as has occurred for many years."—*The Lancet,* April 21st, 1888, p. 768.

SCIENCE DEFINED.　　　Huxley.

RIGHT HON. THOMAS HENRY HUXLEY, M.R.C.S., LL.D., Professor and Dean, Science and Art Department, South Kensington. (V.)

" Common-sense is science exactly in so far as it fulfils the ideal of common-sense ; that is, sees all facts as they are, or, at any rate, without the distortion of prejudice, and reasons from them in accordance with the dictates of sound judgment. And SCIENCE IS SIMPLY COMMON-SENSE AT ITS BEST."—*"The Crayfish"* (London, Kegan Paul & Co., 1880), p. 2.

—— The same.　　　Roscoe.

SIR HENRY ROSCOE, M.P., formerly Professor of Chemistry, Owen's College, Manchester. (P.V.)

" Science is only organised common-sense."—*Speech at the Chemical Society's Jubilee,* " *Times,*" Feb. 26th, 1891.

SCIENCE must not disregard Morality.—*See* MORALITY —Stephen.

SENSITIVENESS of Animals to Pain.—*See* " PAIN IN ANIMALS "—Pritchard.

SILVER, NITRATE OF (Lunar Caustic).　　　Berdoe.

EDWARD BERDOE, M.R.C.S., L.R.C.P.Ed., London. (A.V.)

" This powerful chemical has been largely used in experiments upon animals. It has been very cruelly injected into their veins, causing choking and violent spasms, finally retching, vomiting, and death. Dr. Stillé says, however, that ' there is not the slightest analogy between these effects and those produced on man by its long-continued use.' (*National Dispensatory*, p. 235.)"—*The Futility of Experiments with Drugs on Animals*, by Edward Berdoe (London, 1889), pp. 28, 9.

SNAKE VENOM—Failure of Experiments with.   Fayrer.

SIR JOSEPH FAYRER, K.C.S.I., M.D.Edin., F.R.C.P., F.R.S., Lond. and Edin., etc.   (V.)

"The experiments, of which this is a summary, were commenced in October, 1867, and have been continued as regularly since, at such intervals as time and other and more important avocations permitted. . . . The living creatures experimented on have been the ox, horse, goat, pig, dog, cat, civet, mongoose, rabbit, rat, fowls, kites, herons, fish, innocent snakes, poisonous snakes, lizards, frogs, toads, snails."— "*Summary of Experiments on Snake Poison*," by J. Fayrer, M.D., C.S.I., *Medical Times*, April 1st, 1871, p. 374.

"After careful consideration, fully admitting that in permanganate of potash we have an agent which can chemically neutralize snake-poison, I do not see that more has been done than to draw attention to a local remedy already well known as a chemical antidote, the value of which depends on its efficient application to the contaminated part (which Dr. Wall has pointed out is too uncertain to be reliable). We are still, then, as far off an antidote as ever, and the remarks made by me in 1868 are as applicable now as they were then. They were as follows :—'To conceive of an antidote, as that term is usually understood, we must imagine a substance so subtle as to follow, overtake, and neutralise the venom in the blood, and that shall have the power of counteracting or neutralising the poisonous or deadly influence it has exerted on the vital force. Such a substance has still to be found, nor does our experience of drugs give hopeful anticipations that we shall find it.'"—*Sir J. Fayrer, "Address to Medical Society of London," "British Medical Journal*," Feb. 2nd, 1884.

—— The same—An Antidote for.   "Lancet."

"THE LANCET," Medical Newspaper, London.   (P.V.)

Dr. Mueller, "a country practitioner at the Antipodes, discovered the antidote, and for years practised its use with unfailing success, when Feoktistow, *misled by his experiments*, rejected it. Both published the result of their researches almost synchronously, and Mueller's theory of the action of snake poison, derived from a careful analysis of the symptoms he observed in his patients, was identical in every particular with that drawn by Feoktistow from his splendid and exhaustive experiments. Fully convinced that he had to deal with paresis and paralysis of the motor and vaso-motor nerve centres, and that all symptoms found a ready explanation by this merely functional derangement, Mueller injected the antidote freely, boldly venturing, within less than an hour, on quantities of the drug (strychnine) that would have been fatal but for the antagonism existing between the two poisons. Scores of cases have been placed on record from all parts of Australia.

※   ※   ※   ※   ※

"To explain the causes of failures in the experiments on animals is, in view of the successes on man, scarcely called for. With regard to dogs and cats, it is very evident that their motor nerve centres react very differently from those of man to both snake poison and strychnine. They show greater resistance to the former, for convulsions are not unfrequent at a stage when, in man, paralysis is all but complete."—*The Lancet*, October 4th, 1891, p. 960.

SNAKE VENOM—The Application of the Remedy.   "The Globe."

" THE GLOBE," Evening Newspaper, London. (P.V.)

"The remedy is strychnine. 'It is applied,' he writes, ' by subcutaneous injections of 10 to 20 minims of the liquor strychnine, and continued every 15 minutes until the paralysing effect of the snake venom on the motor and vaso-motor nerve cell is removed, and slight strychnia symptoms supervene. The quantity of the drug required for this purpose depends on the amount of venom imparted by the snake, and may after the bite of a vigorous cobra amount to a grain or more, since more than half a grain has been found necessary to neutralise the effects of the bite of the tiger snake, a reptile much resembling the cobra in appearance, but not imparting nearly as much venom. Strychnine and snake poison being antagonistic in their action, I have found invariably that large doses of strychnine produced no toxic effects in the presence of snake poison, until the action of the latter is completely suspended. These effects, in their initial stage, manifested by slight muscular spasms, are patent to any ordinary observer and perfectly harmless. They pass off quickly, and are an unfailing signal that the antidote is no longer required, and the patient out of danger. Though fully aware of the unfavourable results of experiments with the drug on dogs made at Calcutta and London as well as in Australia, I was, nevertheless, so fully convinced of the correctness of my theory that I administered the antidote fearlessly to persons suffering from snake bite, to a few at the very point of death with pulse at wrists and respiration already suspended, and in every instance with the most gratifying success.' "— *Extract from letter of Dr. Mueller, of Victoria, to Lord Lansdowne, then Viceroy of India, " Globe," Oct. 28th, 1890.*

SODA (Salts of Sodium)—Contradictions of Experiments with.   Berdoe.

EDWARD BERDOE, M.R.C.S., L.R.C.P.Ed., London.   (A.V.)

" The salts of sodium seem to have little influence over the higher animals, but frogs are more susceptible to their action, dying in convulsions after the injection of the drug.—(*Virchow's Archiv*, Bd. xxxiii., p. 507.) As usual, there are contradictions between eminent physiologists as to the action of this medicine upon animals.

" Grandeau (*Robin's Journal de l'Anatomie*, 1864) found that the injection of one hundred and seven grains of the carbonate of sodium into the vein of a dog produced only very slight symptoms, and that thirty-five grains of the nitrate administered in the same way to a rabbit only caused some convulsive movements.—(*Wood*, p. 593.)

" Guttman says that these salts are without influence upon the nerve centres, the peripheral nerves, or the muscles.— (*Wood*, p. 594.)

" According to Guttman (*Virchow's Archiv*, Bd. xxxv.), the Soda salts, when injected into the blood in very large amounts, will slowly cause death, the agony being very prolonged, and, when the chloride is used, convulsions are developed.—(*Wood*, p. 594.)

" Podocaepow says that they do exert a very feeble action upon the peripheral nerves and the muscles.—(*Wood*, p. 594.)" —*The Futility of Experiments with Drugs on Animals*, by Edward Berdoe (London, 1889), pp. 35, 36.

SPINAL CORD, THE.   Brown-Séquard.

CHAS. EDOUARD BROWN-SÉQUARD, M.D. (the late), Coll. de France, Paris.   (V.)

" Experiments upon the medulla oblongata, to decide if the crossing of the conductors of sensitive impressions, coming from the trunk and limbs, has taken place before they reach this organ or not, cannot give positive results, because the reflex movements are so energetic after a section of a lateral half of this nervous centre, that it is very difficult to know the degree of sensibility. But pathological facts observed in man will settle the question."—*Lectures on the Nervous System* (London, 1858).

SPINAL CORD, THE.   Brown-Séquard.

CHAS. EDOUARD BROWN-SÉQUARD, M.D. (the late), Coll. de France, Paris. (V.)

" The question relative to the place of passage in the spinal cord, of the impressions of temperature, and of some other kinds of impressions, cannot be solved by vivisections. But pathological facts observed in man will teach us much more concerning all the sensitive impressions which are not purely painful, than experiments upon animals."—*Lectures on the Nervous System* (London, 1858).

—— The same.   Brown-Séquard.

CHAS. EDOUARD BROWN-SÉQUARD, M.D. (the late), Coll. de France, Paris. (V.)

" It is by far very much more difficult to determine what are the parts of the spinal cord employed in voluntary movements, than to find out what are those through which the sensitive impressions pass. I have long been in doubt in this respect, and even now, after having carefully watched a great many animals, on the spinal cord of which certain alterations had been made, and after having read a great many pathological cases, I still hesitate as regards various points."—*Lectures on the Nervous System* (London, 1858), *Lect.* iv.

—— The same.   Gimson.

W. GIMSON GIMSON, M.D., M.R.C.S., Witham, Essex. (A.V.)

" Sir Astley Cooper made a section of a lateral half of the spinal cord of a dog, and produced a loss of voluntary movements in the corresponding side of the body. Most of the living experimenters agree upon this fact, that such a section causes paralysis only on the side injured. 'I (says Brown-Séquard) have ascertained, a great many times, that this is not perfectly right. There is always, even in mammals, after a transversal section of the whole of a lateral half of the spinal cord, at least some appearance of voluntary movements in the

Q

side of injury, and always also a diminution of voluntary movements in the opposite side." Vivisections show that there is but a slight decussation of the conductors of voluntary movements in the spinal cord in animals, while pathological cases seem to show that there is no decussation of these conductors in this organ in man. Anatomy teaches that the anterior roots send a large part of their fibres transversely across the cord, so that many fibres of the anterior roots of the left side decussate with as many fibres of the anterior roots of the right side. It seems extremely probable that these fibres, or at least many of them, are employed for reflex movements. The teachings of experimentation and of pathology are both opposed to our admitting that these decussating fibres are all voluntary motor conductors.—(*Lect.* iv. and v., 1858.) Nor are we able, speaking at the present time, to say that experimental physiology upon animals has yielded us any more satisfactory conclusion, any 'scientific result' upon this disputed question."—*Vivisections and Painful Experiments on Living Animals: their Unjustifiability* (London, 1879), pp. 38, 39.

SPINAL CORD, THE—Reflex Action.   Gimson.

W. GIMSON GIMSON, M.D., M.R.C.S., Witham, Essex. (A.V.)

"It is by the 'reflex power' of the spinal cord and the medulla oblongata that exist 'the conditions requisite for the maintenance of the various muscular movements which are essential to the continuance of the organic processes'; and, as Dr. Marshall Hall has pointed out, it especially governs the various orifices of ingress and egress.—(*Carpenter*, p. 680.)

　　*　　　　*　　　　*　　　　*　　　　*

"For a long time, the only proofs of independent power of the spinal cord as a nerve centre were derived from the lower animals, and these could not be reconciled with the results of disease or injury of the spinal cord in man (p. 43).

　　　*　　　　*　　　　*　　　　*　　　　*

"It was only by the direction of the attention by Dr. Marshall Hall to pathological observations that light was thrown upon the subject, and the want of analogy explained (p. 44)."—*Vivisections and Painful Experiments on Animals: their Unjustifiability* (London, 1879).

SQUILL—Contradictions of Experiments with.   Berdoe.

EDWARD BERDOE, M.R.C.S., L.R.C.P.Ed., London. (A.V.)

"Everybody knows how valuable this drug is in bronchial

affections; it is, perhaps, the commonest ingredient in a bottle of ordinary cough medicine. Yet, as Dr. Stillé says (p. 1279), in summing up the results of many experiments upon animals with the active principle of squill—*scillitin*—' There is nothing in the results of scientific investigation even to suggest that squill acts upon the bronchial mucous membrane, but the much more direct and conclusive evidence of clinical experience leaves no doubt of its great value in bronchitis.' Some physiologists, quoted by the author of these remarks, killed a number of rabbits by a poisonous dose of the drug; it produced violent inflammation and· erosion of the stomach, and hæmorrhage about the heart, kidneys, brain, and lungs was found: but on the same experiments being repeated by Husemann and Konig no injury of stomach or kidneys was discovered."—*The Futility of Experiments with Drugs on Animals*, by Edward Berdoe (London, 1889), pp. 36, 37.

STRYCHNINE—Uselessness of Experi-   Berdoe. ments with, on Animals.

EDWARD BERDOE, M.R.C.S., L.R.C.P.Ed., London. (A.V.)

" An alkaloid prepared from *Nux Vomica*. This deadly poison, like so many others which we have considered, bears out to the full our contention that it is in vain to attempt to discover the physiological action of drugs on man by experimenting with them upon animals. 'Very minute portions of strychnia in the soil will destroy the life of growing plants.'— (*Stillé, Therapeutics*, p. 1362.)

" Flies and intestinal worms are readily killed by it, and it is very fatal to fish. It is generally believed that the frog is peculiarly sensitive to strychnine, but Falck maintains that in proportion to its weight it is really not so susceptible to its influence as various mammals, and that ' it requires four times the dose needed by dogs, cats, rabbits, etc., to produce an equal effect upon frogs.'—(*Stillé, loc. cit.*) Birds appear to be comparatively insusceptible to its action. Stillé says that a hen, in progressive doses, at last took two and a half drachms of nux vomica daily. It requires ten times as much strychnine to kill a chicken as would suffice for a pheasant. Yet half a drachm of this poison has proved fatal to human beings.— (*Guy and Ferrier's Forensic Medicine*, 4th Ed., p. 572.) The ruminating animals are not so readily affected as other quadrupeds when the poison is taken by the mouth. Ten grains may fail to kill a sheep when thus administered, though half of a grain may kill a man. The same would be fatal to the sheep if administered hypodermically or into the veins. The action of the poison on the goat is similar to that on the sheep. "In whatever way it is given to cats, whether by the stomach, injected into the veins, or under the skin, they 'resist it singularly,' says Stillé. Yet dogs are easily killed by it. It has been enclosed in fulminating bullets to kill whales, and it has been observed that when so poisoned they perish in the spasms which are so characteristic of its action on many other animals, yet 'guinea-pigs and monkeys are said to be comparatively insusceptible to it.'—(*Stillé, loc. cit.*)

"Dr. Lauder-Brunton minutely details the cruel experiments of Majendie on the physiological action of strychnine upon dogs. . . . In page 147 of his *Text Book of Pharmacology*, he states that the strychnine was introduced under the skin of the thigh of a dog; soon the poison began to produce symptoms of general malaise; the poor beast 'took shelter in a corner of the laboratory,' and convulsions of the muscles of the body occurred, 'the fore feet quitting the ground for a moment on account of the sudden extension of the spine.' The animal was quiet for a few seconds, and was then seized with convulsions 'more marked and prolonged than the first.' Others succeeded, gradually becoming more severe. Each time the animal was touched a convulsion immediately followed. . . . No cutting operation could have caused more intense suffering than this injection of strychnine caused the dogs used by Majendie. As for the utility of such experiments Stillé says, *loc. cit.*, 'Although physiological experiments do not lead to the suggestion that strychnine acts upon the peripheral ends of nerves, clinical observation, as in so many other cases, is supposed to demonstrate what the former method has failed to show.'"—*The Futility of Experiments with Drugs on Animals*, by Edward Berdoe (London, 1889), pp. 37–39.

STUDENTS VIVISECTING. Mills.

JAMES B. MILLS, M.R.C.V.S., Military Service (formerly a Student at Edinburgh), a witness before the Royal Commission. (V.)

"Having become a senior, I was introduced to a great number of vivisections, and on some occasions operated myself. The experiments were certainly never designed to discover any new fact, to elucidate any obscure phenomena, but simply to demonstrate the most ordinary facts of physiology. Our victims were sometimes dogs, but more frequently cats. Many of the latter were caught by means of a poisoned bait, the animal being secured while suffering from the agonies caused by the poison, when antidotes were applied for their restoration. They were then imprisoned in a cupboard at the students' lodgings, and kept there until a meeting could be arranged. Sometimes the students secured their victims by what is known as a cat hunt ; that is, a raid on cats by students armed with sticks late at night. I am not prepared to say that the object of the students was to commit cruelty, or that there was any morbid desire to witness pain, but I say emphatically that there was reckless love of experimentation. What, for instance, could justify the following experiment, performed for the purpose of witnessing the action of a cat's heart? The operator first of all made an incision through the skin of the animal's chest. The skin was then laid back by hooks, in order to enable the operator to cut through the cartilage of the breast-bone, and to draw his knife across the ribs for the purpose of nicking them. This process is necessary to enable him to snap the ribs and lay the fractured part back. . . . In a few cases the animals were narcotised." He exonerates the professor from knowledge of the above.—*Evid. Roy. Com.* (London, 1876). Q. 1687.

When Mr. Mills appeared himself later on, before the Commissioners, he confirmed the above statement, which had been signed by him, and added that he had information that "last session (*i.e.* 1874-5) the practice of vivisection among the students continued," and gave the following particulars (Q. 4957): "Last winter the subject that was operated on was a horse, and it was bought for the purpose of dissection. This animal was subjected during a whole week to operations, such as tenotomy and neurotomy, and various minor operations." (No chloroform being given.) (Q. 4970): " . . . Were animals bought and operated upon simply for the purpose of exhibition and demonstration? "—"They were." (Q. 4971): "In the college?"—"They were." (Q. 4972): "That was so when you were a student in the college, was it?"—"Yes." (Q. 4975): "Now what animals were operated upon simply for the purpose of demonstration?"—"Horses and donkeys" (Q. 4981) "and dogs." (Q. 5055. Questioned as to private experiments): "A few of the medical college students were always mixed with the veterinary students." Question 5073 and following questions elicited also the statement that he, himself, opened the chest of a cat, in private lodging, without giving chloroform. The cat lived seven or eight minutes. The object was to see the heart beat, but the remaining vivisections were simply for dissecting out nerves, and yet the animal was alive.—*See Evid. Roy. Com.* (London, 1876).

The Principal of the College, Mr. Williams, was subsequently questioned as to the horse mentioned by Mr. Mills being kept for a week. (Q. 6027) : " The result of your inquiry is that you do believe the thing was done ? "—" Yes." He goes on to explain that he was not aware at the time of this case. Mr. Williams was then asked (Q 6033): " Were those operations performed under chloroform ? "—" No." " Were no anæsthetics given ? "—" No, none whatever." " Were they painful operations ? "—" Very. The animal was cast by means of hobbles."—" And were the operations chiefly on the nerves ?" —" Nerves and tendons." [The above was, Mr. Williams stated, against rules, but students were allowed to bleed a horse, while it waited to be killed, without superintendence.]—*Evid. Roy. Com.* (London. 1876).

SURGERY AND VIVISECTION.   "Lancet."

" THE LANCET," Medical Newspaper, London.   (P.V.)

" Vivisection has undoubtedly tended to advance the art of medicine ; but it is equally true that mankind has had to find out for itself what surgery it could bear.   The great triumphs of surgery have been made independently of it."—*The Lancet,* Aug. 25th, 1894, p. 446.

TARTAR EMETIC—Contradictions of   Berdoe.
   Experiments with.

EDWARD BERDOE, M.R C.S., L.R.C.P.Ed., London.   (A.V.)

" Many cruel experiments have been performed upon animals with this drug.   It seems to have been proved in this instance that its action is precisely the same on the lower animals as on man.—(*See Wood's Therapeutics,* p. 151.)   In contradiction to this statement, Dr. Lauder-Brunton says that ' Ipecacuanha, or Tartar Emetic, will cause vomiting in man, but does not do o in rabbits.   The reason of this is that the position of the stomach in the rabbit is different from that in man, and is such that the animal cannot vomit.'—(*Pharmacology,* p. 40.) Nöbiling had a theory that the action of tartar emetic upon the heart is owing to the potash it contains.   He performed a number of experiments to support his theory, and another experimenter (*Wood,* p. 151) says, ' This theory in itself is so improbable that it would seem scarcely worthy of discussion were it not for the fact that Nöbiling asserts that the tartarate of antimony and soda is not poisonous.'   ' Dr. Radziejewski (*Reichert's Archiv für Anatomie,* 1871) has repeated and extended the experiments of Nöbiling, and completely disproved both the asserted fact and the theory based upon it.'—(*Wood*, p. 151.")—*The Futility of Experiments with Drugs on Animals*, by Edward Berdoe (London, 1889), pp. 39, 40.

TEACHING—Vivisection not Necessary for.   Tait.

LAWSON TAIT, F.R.C.S., late Professor of Gynæcology, Queen's College, Birmingham. (A.V.)

" I have a little bit of information that I think will please you. I happen to be a member of the council of our large Science College at Birmingham, and also one of the council of the Medical School, and some seven or eight years ago the Professors of Physiology appealed to the Council for permission to apply to the Home Secretary for a licence to practise Vivisection ; we took the matter very carefully into consideration, and the council decided that no permission would be given to any kind of experiments on living animals within the walls of the Institution. Our decision was considered by some as a very disadvantageous one to arrive at, as it would drive away our medical students. Now I want to tell you this. At that time, that is six or seven years ago, we had about 110 or 120 students ; at the present time, now that we have absolutely prohibited the use of those experiments, we have more than double that number. With this I think you will see that Vivisection is unnecessary for teaching purposes, as our students have carried off just as many prizes as any students elsewhere."—*Speech at the Annual Meeting of the London Society*, *St. James's Hall, May 26th, 1891.*

TETANUS.   Various Authors.

" According to the Pasteurian theory tetanus is incurable once it shows itself."—" *Daily News'* " *Paris Correspondent*, Oct. 25th, 1894.

" Its prophylaxy resides before all else in the application of the aseptic or antiseptic method. Equally with the infection purulent, as in the case of erysipelas, tetanus is a malady resulting from uncleanness. It is necessary then, when one finds himself in presence of a wound, however small it may be— since even superficial wounds give rise to tetanus—not to abandon it to itself, but to close it."—*Dr Cabanès in Journal de Médecine de Paris*, Aug. 13th, 1893, p. 395.

" The most rigorous antisepticism is, according to my observation, the procedure the most certain to arrest the propagation of the malady."—*M. Verneuil at Academy of Medicine of Paris*, " *Figaro*," July 5th, 1893.

" In man, some cases of insidious tetanus have been, according to Tizzoni and Cantani, cured by the serum, but it is probable that these cases would have got well without any special treatment."—*M. Berger, Surgeon, at Academy of Medicine, Paris*, " *Medical Press and Circular*," *Paris correspondence*, June 7th, 1893.

TETANUS—Duration of Immunity.   " The Lancet."

"THE LANCET," Medical Newspaper, London. (P.V.)

" The experiments and results refer to tetanus only. In testing the duration of the immunity afforded by serum from various sources it was found that in rabbits treated with horse-serum the immunity was lost in sixteen days, and that there was rather strong local reaction. In rabbits treated with dog-serum the immunity vanished in fifteen days, and again there was considerable local reaction. In rabbits treated with rabbit-serum there was but slight local reaction, and the immunity was prolonged to twenty-one days. In the experiments the various kinds of serum injected were of the same immunising power, or were carefully made so by using proportional doses."—" *The Lancet*," *Berlin correspondence*, Jan. 13th, 1894, p. 125.

—— The same—Death from,   " Medical after Inoculation.   Journal."

"THE BRITISH MEDICAL JOURNAL," Organ of the British Medical Association, London. (P.V.)

" L. T., aged 38, trod on a nail on May 8th; four days later he had 'rheumatism' in the ankle and wrist of the same side. On May 16th he complained of much stiffness in the neck and back, and was unable to open his mouth or swallow; later in the day he was admitted into the Norfolk and Norwich Hospital. He had a small scar on the sole of the left foot. He suffered from constant opisthotonos, and during the two next days he had five spasms, during which respiration ceased, and the face became blue. His temperature rose to 101°, the pulse varied from 78 to 90, and was weak. Professor Roux had already been kind enough to supply us with the amount of anti-toxin required for the treatment of a single case; the whole of this was injected hypodermically under chloroform in four equal doses. The first administration was made on the evening of May 6th, it was repeated every six hours without appreciable effect, the patient dying in a spasm on the evening of the 17th."—*Case reported by* Dr. F. W. Burton-Fanning, *Norfolk and Norwich Hospital, in " British Medical Journal,"* Sept. 29th, 1894, p. 725.

THEIN (from Tea)—Contradictions of Experimenters as to.

Berdoe.

EDWARD BERDOE, M.R.C.S., L.R.C.P.Ed., London.   (A.V.)

" Chemists and physiologists tell us that the active principle of tea, *Thein*, and that of coffee. *Caffein*, are identical.   Dr. A. Burnett experimented with these alkaloids upon frogs, mice, rabbits, and cats, and came to the conclusion that they were ' identical throughout the whole range of their action.'   Are we to conclude, therefore, that the action of tea and coffee on the human system is identical ?   By no means.   Says Stillé (p. 1424), ' The identity of these alkaloids in their physiology does not imply a similar identity in tea and coffee.   As little should we be entitled to infer that all alcoholic drinks produce identical effects because they all contain alcohol as their chief constituent.   It is just as certain that tea and coffee differ in their action upon the human system as that Rhenish or Bordeaux wines act very differently from whisky or brandy, although in all of these liquors the common cause of their effects is alcohol.'   So much, therefore, for the value of physiological medicine."—*The Futility of Experiments with Drugs on Animals*, by Edward Berdoe (London, 1889), p. 40.

THERAPEUTICS AND RESEARCH.   " Medical Journal."

"THE BRITISH MEDICAL JOURNAL," Organ of the British Medical Association, London.   (P.V.)

" During the last thirty years the experimental researches of pharmacologists have accumulated a large number of more or less isolated facts regarding the influence of the chemical constitution of substances on their physiological action.   The subject has attracted able investigators in every civilised country, and although recently progress has been more rapid, and some practical benefit has resulted to the art of healing, yet on taking a wide view of the whole question it must be admitted that little more has been accomplished than to break ground here and there.   Our accumulated knowledge is not yet sufficient to enable us to formulate any general laws governing the relationship, and practical value to clinical medicine of all the labour expended is seen only in a few directions. . . . We are completely ignorant of the chemical structure of the whole class of cardiac tonics—in fact, in many cases the active principle has never been obtained pure from the crude drug. It seems certain that some of these are much less cumulative and dangerous than others, but until we know on what differences in chemical constitution their physiological peculiarities depend it is unlikely that any advances of permanent value will be obtained. The same is true of purgative medicines. By experience we have acquired a considerable amount of empirical skill in the use of both classes of remedies; but more than this we can scarcely claim—certainly not a high degree of scientific knowledge."—*British Medical Journal*, Jan. 27th, 1894, pp. 201-2.

THYROID INOCULATIONS.   Fox.

R. HINGSTON FOX, M.D.Brux., M.R.C.P.Lond., M.R.C.S., etc., London. (P.V.)

" The want of constancy complained of in the therapeutical effects of the gland may be due to variations in the gland itself. I have satisfied myself that such variations occur by personal observation. It is impossible, therefore, to assert that one gland is equivalent to any other, either in size or quality. . . . Not until chemists succeed in isolating and identifying the active principle to which thyroid gland owes its remarkable physiological effects, can we hope to obtain any uniformity in physiological or therapeutical effects. In the meantime our experiments must remain more or less rough and, therefore, open to many fallacies and discrepancies."—*Speech at the Medical Society of London*, Jan. 8th, "*Medical Week*," Jan. 12th, 1894.

—— **The same.**—*See also* MYXŒDEMA.

TOBACCO—Irreconcilable Results of   Berdoe.
   Experiments with.

EDWARD BERDOE, M.R.C.S., L.R.C.P.Ed., London. (A.V.)

" The active principle of this plant is nicotia, and it stands next to prussic acid in the rapidity and energy of its poisonous action. Tobacco is poisonous to all forms of life, yet ' herbivorous animals are not readily affected by it.'—(*Stillé*, p. 1406). Many experimenters have investigated its action on the nerves, muscular system, and circulation of the lesser animals, chief of whom are Traube and Rosenthal: but Wood says, p. 363, 'that the results obtained by Rosenthal are difficult to reconcile with the effects—already quoted from Traube.'"— *The Futility of Experiments with Drugs on Animals* (London, 1889). p. 41.

TOOT PLANT OF AUSTRALIA (Coriaria   Berdoe. Sarmentosa)—Varying Effects of, on Men and Animals.

EDWARD BERDOE, M.R.C.S., L.R.C.P.Ed., London.   (A.V.)

"This plant is exceedingly poisonous to human beings, yet native horses and cattle, and it is said even 'old colonists,' eat the plant with tolerable impunity. Fifteen berries of another species (*C. Myrtifolia*) have caused the death of an adult. A teaspoonful of an extract of the juice will kill a cat in two hours; yet when the plant is given to rabbits they do not appear to be affected by it.—(*Woodman & Tidy's Toxicology*, p. 392.)"—*The Futility of Experiments with Drugs on Animals*, by Edward Berdoe (London, 1889), p. 41.

TRANSFUSION.   Tait.

LAWSON TAIT, F.R.C.S., late Professor of Gynæcology, Queen's College, Birmingham. (A.V.)

"This operation was not initiated, as asserted by Mr· Gamgee, in the second half of the seventeenth century by Dr. Lower, of Oxford, nor was it first proposed as a legitimate surgical operation at all. It was proposed, and in all probability was really practised, by the alchemists of the sixteenth century as an attempt to obtain for the wealthy aged a renewal of their lease of life, after the theory and legend of Faustus. Certain it is that allusions to it are frequent, though the first actual account of its performance is given by André Libavius, Professor of Medicine at Halle (Helmst. 1602), as having been performed by him in 1594, the blood of a young healthy man being transfused into a man aged and decrepit, but able and willing to pay for the supposed advantage. In the early part of the seventeenth century it was a good deal discussed from this point of view, forgotten for a while, and then after the Restoration it was reconsidered, and a great deal written about it in this country and on the Continent.

    ✻   ✻   ✻   ✻   ✻

"The scheme of transfusion in all the experiments of the seventeenth-century descriptions which I have seen was to

take arterial blood from an animal and pass it into the veins of
another, and that this was successful is not surprising.   But
this has never been attempted in modern times upon man.   It
certainly would not be justifiable; because, to interfere with a
large artery—and a large artery would be required—in a man
is always an extremely risky thing.   Dr. Lower, who is Mr.
Gamgee's authority, in 1667 injected, or tried to inject, arterial
blood from a lamb into a man; but the operation was so badly
done that I do not believe any blood really passed.   Mr. Flint
South gives a succinct history of the matter, and tells us that
it was revived by the plan of mediate transfusion in the early
part of the present century.   The former experiments were
fruitlessly repeated and others tried.   The result is that the
operation has a very insecure hold on professional opinion.   I
have seen it performed seven times without success in a single
instance.   I have twice been asked to do it, and have declined,
and both patients are now alive and well.   We hear a great
deal of cases in which patients have survived after transfusion
has been performed, but we hear little or nothing of its
failures.   Personally, I have no confidence in the proceeding."
—*Uselessness of Vivisection*, by L. Tait (Birmingham, 1882),
pp. 24-26.

TRIMETHYLAMINA—Cruelties and Con-   Berdoe.
  tradictions of Experimenters with.

EDWARD BERDOE, M.R.C.S., L.R.C.P.Ed., London.   (A.V.)

"This drug was first employed medicinally for the cure of
articular rheumatism in 1854.   It is obtained by distilling
herring brine or stale fish with lime.   Injected under a rabbit's
skin it caused trembling, convulsive movements, agitation,
increased sensibility and quickening of the breathing and
heart's action—then depression or collapse, paralysis, and
death by asphyxia, in fact, such symptoms as were termed by
Mr. Erichsen (the late Inspector) in his report as consequent
upon ' hypodermic injections ' and 'mostly of a painless character.'   To dogs the drug was given by the mouth, producing
vomiting, anxiety, distress, immobility, muscular tremors,
emaciation, bloody urine at the end of six days.   (Note the
length of time occupied by these injection experiments, and the
pain and extreme misery inflicted on the animals.)   When the
rabbits were killed by the injections, mortification was found
at the point of the insertion of the needle, the lungs and
kidneys were congested; yet all these things we are told are
painless and trifling because they do not involve vivisection in

the ordinary sense. Husemann, Dujardin-Beaumetz, and Stillé, are at variance as to the physiological action of the drug. Its action upon man appears to be quite different from the effects observed on the rabbits, and it has been entirely superseded as a remedy for rheumatism by the salicylates, so that the sufferings of the animals have not in this instance conferred any boon on medicine."—*The Futility of Experiments with Drugs on Animals*, by Edward Berdoe (London, 1889), pp. 41-42.

TUBERCULOSIS—Uselessness of Inoculation for.　　　　　　　　　Koch.

ROBERT KOCH, M.D., Berlin.　(V.)

" You saw the dog which was injected with a minimum quantity of tubercle bacilli. The injection was made in the abdominal cavity, and produced an exquisite tubercular peritonitis. Nevertheless, the dog finally recovered entirely, and seemed perfectly well. Then the same dog was used again, and a large number of bacilli were introduced into the abdominal cavity. You will see that the dog is fatally ill. Now, if one attack conferred immunity, it ought to have been impossible to produce this second attack. Hence I do not think it possible to prevent the disease in that way, nor do I think it necessary to try it."—" *Dr. Robert Koch interviewed*," " *Medical Times*," Aug. 26th, 1882, p. 255.

—— Unproductiveness of Discovery of Microbe of.　　　　　Dowdeswell.

GEORGE FRANCIS DOWDESWELL, M.A., F.R.S., etc. (the late).　(V.)

" It has been lately said by a most eminent authority in medicine and pharmacology, in relation to the action of bacteria, that the future of medicine will be rather preventive than remedial; but experience as yet goes to show that this consummation must be rather due to general measures of sanitation than to any conclusion founded upon ætiological or microscopical investigation. This disappointed expectation is strikingly exemplified in the circumstance that the demonstration by Koch of the micro-parasite of tuberculosis—which discovery has been characterized as one of the greatest achievements in medical science of the present age—has been utterly unproductive of the very smallest improvement in the treatment of the most dire disease prevalent in this country. Beyond that, too,

the result of experiments upon the lower animals is directly at variance both with clinical observation and daily experience."
—*The Lancet*, April 21st, 1888.

TUBERCULOSIS—Effects of Inoculation, Animals and Man. Koch.

ROBERT KOCH, M.D., Professor, Berlin. (V.)

"As regards the effect of the remedy on human beings, it was evident at the very beginning of the experiments that in one very important point the effect of the remedy on man is entirely different from that on the guinea-pig, which is the animal usually experimented upon. Here again is a fresh and conclusive proof of that most important rule for all experimentalists, that an experiment on an animal gives no certain indication of the result of the same experiment upon a human being. Human beings showed themselves to be very much more susceptible to the effects of the remedy than the guinea-pig. As much as two cubic centimètres, and even more, of the non-diluted liquid can be injected under the skin of a healthy guinea-pig without any noticeable injury to it. But for a healthy grown-up man 0·25 cubic centimètre sufficed to produce a very intense effect. Calculating by body weight, therefore, the 1500th part of the quantity which produces no visible effect on the guinea-pig has a very powerful effect on the human being."—*From "The Cure of Consumption," by Prof. Robert Koch, authorised translation (London, Heinemann, 1890), pp. 8-9.*

—— The same.—*See* "Koch, Latest Medical Verdict on."

—— The same—False Hopes. "Blackwood's Magazine."

" BLACKWOOD'S MAGAZINE," Edinburgh. (N.)

" He roused a frantic hope in the bosoms of sufferers all over the world, and of those who loved them. He caused such excitement as has rarely been known before, both among the learned and the ignorant. And then it all came to nothing. The disappointment, the disillusion, was immense; and as a matter of fact, from standing out against the sky as one of the great benefactors of the human race—as he did for some time, with all sorts of substantial rewards and honours prematurely bestowed—the figure of Koch has disappeared altogether, to be hailed by nothing but a grin or a groan, according to the disposition of the spectator, should it make any furtive appearance again.—*Blackwood's Magazine,* Jan. 1895.

TUBERCULOSIS—Experimenter Poisoned by Germs of. "Gaulois."

"THE GAULOIS," Paris Newspaper. (P.V.)

" M. Jules Chabry, M.D., sub-chief of service at the Pasteur Institute, died yesterday, after a lengthened illness, of tuberculosis (consumption) contracted in a laboratory in studying bacteriological problems."—"*The Gaulois*," Nov. 26th, 1893. *(Also published in " L'Intransigeant,*" Nov. 28th.)*

UNCERTAINTY of Result of Experiments. Leffingwell.

ALBERT LEFFINGWELL, M.D., Cambridge, Mass., U.S.A. (R.)

" One danger to which scientific truth seems to be exposed is a peculiar tendency to under-estimate the numberless uncertainties and contradictions created by experimentation upon living beings. Judging from the enthusiasm of its advocates, one would think that by this method of interrogating nature all fallacies can be detected, all doubts determined. But, on the contrary, the result of experimentation, in many directions, is to plunge the observer into the abyss of uncertainty. Take, for example, one of the simplest and yet most important questions possible—the degree of sensibility in the lower animals. Has an infinite number of experiments enabled physiologists to determine for us the mere question of pain ? Suppose an amateur experimenter in London, desirous of performing some severe operations upon frogs, to hesitate because of the extreme painfulness of his methods, what replies would he be likely to obtain from the highest scientific authorities of England as to the sensibility of these creatures ? We may fairly judge their probable answers to such inquiries from their evidence already given before a Royal Commission."—" *Vivisection,*" " *Lippincott's Magazine,*" Aug., 1884, pp. 126, 127.

—— The same.—*See* RESPIRATION—BARLOW.

UREA. Berdoe.

EDWARD BERDOE, M.R.C.S., L.R.C.P.Ed., London. (A.V.)

" Ségalas demonstrated that urea injected into the veins of animals notably increased the discharge of urine. According to Rabateau it exhibits no diuretic action in human beings, even in very large doses."—*The Futility of Experiments with Drugs on Animals.* by Edward Berdoe (London, 1889), p. 42.

USELESSNESS OF VIVISECTION.   De Sinety.

LOUIS DE SINETY, M.D., fo merly Prof. of General Anatomy
at the Medical Faculty, Paris. (V.)

" I have myself made a fair number of experiments relative
to the innervation of the mammary glands on female guinea-
pigs. . . . Considering the contradictory results, it would
be well to describe the experiments before arriving at any
conclusions. . . . Experiment No. 1, June 10th, 1874.—
Guinea-pig in lactation. The mammary nerve on one side is
laid bare, and insulated by means of a thread. The animal
exhibits signs of acute pain, especially when the nerve is stimulated by an electric current ; but the stimulation, prolonged
during ten minutes, produces no appreciable effect on the teats
or on the amount of milk secreted. I divided the nerve, and
on the following day, June 11th, there was as much milk in one
gland as in the other ; nor did the electric stimulation re-applied
to both ends of the divided nerve produce any apparent effect
on the glandular function. . . . I have selected these five
experiments from those I had noted down in my book, as I
made them under varying conditions. In all of them the results
were negative. . . . Roehrig observed that in the goat the
effects were different—as M. Lafont had said—which proves
once more that the conclusions arrived at must not be general-
ized, and that the phenomena may vary considerably according
to the species of animal."—" De l'Innervation de la Mamelle,"
Report de la Soc. de Biologie, October 25th, 1879, " Gaz. Méd. de
Paris," 1879, p. 593.

——— The same.   Smith.

FRED A. A. SMITH, M.D., Cheltenham. (A.V.)

" Some five-and-twenty years ago, as a student, being fond of
all kinds of experiments, and being especially fond of physiological research, I often witnessed and sometimes performed
vivisections ; but I soon found out that little or no good ever
came from such proceedings. As my mind became more
mature, I became convinced that the whole thing was wrong,
and that as Christian and civilized people we have no moral
right to inflict needless pain upon any of the lower animals
for our benefit, whatever that benefit may be ; and I at once,
as a medical man of many years' standing, declare that little
or nothing has been found out by the aforesaid experiments to
warrant their continuance any longer, and sincerely hope that
at any rate they will be discontinued in this our country. I
am proud to enrol myself among your society."—Letter to Miss
Wakeman, dated Feb. 10th, 1888.

USELESSNESS OF VIVISECTION.　Crisp.

EDWARDS CRISP, M.D. (the late), Witness before Royal Commission, 1875. (A.V.)

"I am rather a penitent upon this question. I have been a vivisector for some time. For several years I cut into animals, removing their spleens, and the thyroid glands (the glands in the neck), and performed many other experiments, and as I advanced in age, and I hope in wisdom, I saw fit to alter many opinions that I had formed at an earlier period; and I have come to the conclusion that vivisection as practised, especially on the Continent, has not led to the good that its advocates believe. I think that there are many false inferences drawn."—*Evid. Roy. Com.* (London, 1876), Q. 6,157.

—— The same.　Fergusson.

SIR WILLIAM FERGUSSON. Bart., F.R.S. (the late), Sergeant Surgeon to the Queen (born 1808 ; died 1877). (A.V.)

"The impression on my mind is, that these experiments are done frequently in a most reckless manner, (Q. 1,036) and (if known to the public) would bring the reputation of certain scientific men far below what it should be. (1,037) I have reason to imagine that sufferings incidental to such operations are protracted in a very shocking manner. I will give you an illustration of an animal being crucified for several days, perhaps introduced several times in a lecture-room for the class to see how the experiment was going on. (1,028) I believe it (the above) to be done in this country. Mr. Syme lived to express an abhorrence of such operations, at all events if they were not useful. (1,029) His ultimate authority was strongly on the other side (against them), as expressed in a special report of his own. (1,030) No man perhaps has ever had more experience of the human subject than Mr. Syme, and I myself have a strong opinion that such an expression, coming from Mr. Syme, was a mature and valuable opinion."—*Evid. Roy. Com.* (London, 1876).

—— The same.　Macaulay.

JAMES MACAULAY, M.A., M.D., F.R.C.S.Ed., London. (A.V.)

"The whole history of this branch of physiological research —from the time of Herophilus, Erasistratus, and the Egyptian operators who had living human bodies to experiment upon, down to our own day, when Professor Ferrier has to be content

R

with the anthropoid progenitor of the human race, and Professor Rutherford with man's faithful dependent, the dog, as the
subjects for examination—the whole history of vivisection, if it
does not convince men of science of the entire uselessness of
these modes of research, will at least force them to admit that
they are of infinitely less service than it is now the custom to
represent them.

  *   *   *   *   *

"A few conclusions, indeed, are given by experimenters as
having been placed by them beyond the reach of controversy;
but these few, I maintain, could have been as surely arrived at
by anatomical and pathological research."—*Vivisection: A
Prize Essay* (London, 1881), pp. 70, 71.

USELESSNESS OF VIVISECTION.   Bowie.

JOHN BOWIE, L.R.C.P., L.R.C.S., Edinburgh. (A.V.)

" Human vivisection is spoken of by Galen as having been
fashionable hundreds of years before his day. He mentions
particularly two celebrated anatomists, Herophilus and Erasistratus, as possessing a more accurate knowledge of the human
organism than all other physicians, surgeons, and physiologists
who lived prior to his time. History testifies to the doleful
fact that these two physiologists alone dissected no fewer than
600 living men and women. Ptolemy Philadelphus was the
name of the tyrant sovereign who handed over from time
to time, through a series of years, the wretched victims for
physiological demonstration. Celsus, writing on this very
theme, says, 'they procured criminals out of prison by Royal
Commission, and dissecting them alive, contemplated while
they were yet breathing what nature had before concealed,
examining their position, figure, colour, size, hardness,
smoothness, and roughness,' etc.

  *   *   *   *   *

"The knowledge of this fact by the Professor (Rutherford),
although it refutes his ascription to Galen as the first to
initiate experiments on animals, may prove of immense value
to him, when he pleads the necessity for hospital patients being
given over for vivisectional enterprise as indispensable to
perfect and complete scientific investigations. How could
such proceedings bring anything else but the degradation and
downfall of the art and practice of medicine."—*Reply to Dr.
Rutherford*, Dec. 24th, 1880 (*Review* Office, 20, St. Giles' Street,
Edinburgh), p. 5.

USELESSNESS OF VIVISECTION— Fletcher.
and Non-necessity.

JOHN FLETCHER, M.D., formerly Lecturer on Physiology and Medical Jurisprudence, Edinburgh Medical School. (A.V.)

"None of the functions of animals need be seen in action in order to be perfectly well understood; they may be abundantly well fancied from preparations and representations of the organs engaged in performing them; and none, certainly, will be exhibited in action in the present lectures. During many years' experience in lecturing on this subject, and in delivering courses of more than ten or twelve times the duration proposed at present, I have never yet found it necessary, in a single instance, to expose a suffering animal, even to students of medicine (who are necessarily, in some degree, familiarized with sights of horror), for the purpose of elucidating any point of physiology, and I certainly shall not begin now; nor can I refrain from stating my belief that experiments on living animals are much less necessary, even to the advancement of this science, than has been sometimes imagined."—*Introductory Lecture (quoted in Dr. Jas. Macaulay's Essay)* (London, 1881), pp. 11, 12.

—— The same. Gimson.

W. GIMSON GIMSON, M.D., M.R.C.S., Witham, Essex. (A.V.)

"It is not by experiments performed on healthy animals that we can hope to gain sound knowledge in the treatment of diseases of the circulating system in man. Hunter's operation for aneurism was the result of reasoning and experience; disease had already proved what Sir Astley Cooper sought to prove by experiments on dogs; and our knowledge gained by the practice of surgery has proved that the lower limb could be adequately supplied with blood after ligation of its main artery."—*Vivisections and Painful Experiments on Animals; their Unjustifiability* (London, 1879), p. 19.

—— The same. Tait.

LAWSON TAIT, F.R.C.S., late Professor of Gynæcology, Queen's College, Birmingham. (A.V.)

"I have given a great deal of attention for many years to this subject, and the more I know of it the more I become satisfied that nothing whatever has been gained by vivisection. Its advocates say that by its means Harvey discovered the circulation of the blood, but the circulation of the blood was dis

covered sixty years before by the dissection of the dead body,
and could have been demonstrated beyond dispute by the
simple expedient of injecting the arteries with coloured size.
Hunter is said to have discovered his cure for aneurism by
vivisection ; but Sir Everard Home clearly shows that it was
by pathological investigation that this was made.   Spencer
Wells claims to have advanced ovariotomy by this means, but
his statements have been blown to the winds by every one of
experience, and all that was established for him was that he
had sacrificed some rabbits to prove a point which had been
settled long before, and had never been disputed.   We are told
that the functions of the posterior roots of the spinal nerves
were discovered by vivisection ; but disease has made far more
accurate experiments, and had done so before, only we were
blind to the lessons.   The only localized function of the brain
which can be accepted as definitely ascertained has been
indicated by disease, and not by experiment.   In fact, every
illustration which the advocates of vivisection put forth falls to
pieces when carefully examined, and those who know most
about it are least in favour of it.   Let us ask who has done
most in this country for natural science, and the answer will
be, Charles Darwin, a man who never in his life did a cruelty,
whose whole nature is gentleness.   I do not say that vivisection may not yet be shown to be necessary, but I do say that
it is not yet so shown."—*Letter, signed " Biologist," in the " Birmingham Daily Post,"* Nov. 23rd, 1881.

USELESSNESS OF VIVISECTION—   Tait.
and Non-necessity.

LAWSON TAIT, F.R.C.S., late Professor of Gynæcology, Queen's
    College, Birmingham.   (A.V.)

" Like every member of my profession, I was brought up in
the belief that by vivisection had been obtained almost every
important fact in physiology, and that many of our most valued
means of saving life and diminishing suffering had resulted
from experiments on the lower animals.   I now know that
nothing of the sort is true concerning the art of surgery ; and not
only do I not believe that vivisection has helped the surgeon
one bit, but I know that it has often led him astray."—*Letter in
" Birmingham Daily Post,"* Dec. 12th, 1884.

—— The same.   .   Taylor.

CHARLES BELL-TAYLOR, M.D., F.R.C.S.Ed., M.R.C.S.Eng.,
    Oculist and Surgeon, Nottingham.   (A.V.)

" Very few men were called upon to operate more frequently

than himself. If this practice were necessary to acquire skill in operating, it would have been necessary for himself, and he could only say that he never vivisected an animal's eye in his life. He knew that his old teacher Syme—certainly one of the first surgeons the world had ever seen—was vehemently opposed to it ; so was the late Sir William Fergusson, Sergeant-Surgeon to the Queen. So he thought they might safely conclude that vivisection was not necessary to the education of a surgeon. Was it necessary for a physician ? Sir Thomas Watson, who had been the leading Metropolitan physician for about half a century, told them that he never saw a vivisectional experiment in his life, and it was a fact that ninety-five per cent. of the general practitioners in this country are entirely innocent of the practice. . . . And he spoke the simple truth. Not only was vivisection devoid of good results, but it had exercised a terribly sinister influence in diverting men s minds from legitimate paths of study. Those paths were at the bedside and the pathological theatre."—*Speech before Nottingham Phil. and Hist. Society*, 1879.

USELESSNESS OF VIVISECTION—and Non-necessity.—
See also DOUBTFUL RESULTS and DROWNING.

—— **The same.** **Foster.**

MICHAEL FOSTER, M.D., F.R.S., Professor of Physiology, University of Cambridge. (V.)

"You do not want much physiology for an understanding of the principles of medicine and of the nature of disease." (p. 783, col. 1.)

    *   *   *   *   *

"Nothing is to my mind more dangerous than the practice of taking, so to speak, 'raw' physiology at once into clinical work ; and if you look back on the history of the profession you will find that these attempts to take physiology straight off into practical use have proved delusive, and to my mind a great deal of discredit has been thrown upon physiology by these attempts."—*From an Address before the Medical Society of University College, London, on the question, "Why should Medical Students Study Physiology ?"—The Lancet*, Oct. 19th, 1889.

—— **The same.** **Huxley.**

THOMAS HENRY HUXLEY, M.R.C.S., LL.D., Professor and Dean, Science and Art Department, South Kensington. (V.)

In the course of a discussion in *The Times* on the subject of

" Political Ethics "—the ethics of land-acquisition and land-owning, and Mr. Herbert Spencer's views in relation thereto —Mr. Spencer wrote:—" ' Your treatment is quite at variance with physiological principles ' would probably be the criticism passed by a modern practitioner on the doings of a Sangrado, if we supposed one to have survived. 'Oh, bother your physiological principles,' might be the reply. ' I have got to cure this disease, and my experience tells me that bleeding and frequent draughts of hot water are needed.' ' Well,' would be the rejoinder, ' if you do not kill your patient, you will at any rate greatly retard his recovery, as you would probably be aware had you read Professor Huxley's *Lessons on Elementary Physiology* and the more elaborate books on the subject which medical students have to master.' This imaginary conversation will sufficiently suggest that, before there can be rational treatment of a disordered state of the bodily functions, there must be a conception of what constitutes their ordered state : knowing what is abnormal implies knowing what is normal. That Professor Huxley recognises this truth is, I suppose, proved by the inclusion of physiology in that course of medical education which he advocates. If he says that abandonment of the Sangrado treatment was due, not to the teachings of physiology, but to knowledge empirically gained, then I reply that if he expands this statement so as to cover all improvements in medical treatment he suicidally rejects the teaching of physiological principles as useless."—*Times*, November 15th, 1889.

To this appeal, Professor Huxley replied in these terms :— " Mr. Spencer addresses a sort of *argumentum ad hominem* to me. It is hardly chosen with so much prudence as might have been expected. Mr. Spencer assumes that in the present state of physiological and medical science, the practitioner would be well advised who should treat his patients by deduction from physiological principles ('absolute physiological therapeutics,' let us say) rather than by careful induction from the observed phenomena of disease and of the effects of medicines. Well, all I can reply is, Heaven forbid that I should ever fall into that practitioner's hands ; and if I thought any writings of mine could afford the smallest pretext for the amount of manslaughter of which that man would be guilty, I should be grieved indeed. Mr. Spencer could not have chosen a better illustration of the gulf fixed between his way of thinking and mine. Whenever physiology (including pathology), pharmacy and hygiene, are perfect sciences, I have no doubt that the practice of medicine will be deducible from the first principles of these sciences. That happy day has not arrived yet, and I fancy it is not likely to arrive for some time."— *Times*, November 18th, 1889.

USELESSNESS OF VIVISECTION in curing Disease.

Leffingwell.

ALBERT LEFFINGWELL, M.D., Cambridge, Mass., U.S.A. (R.)

" Has physiological experimentation during the last quarter of a century contributed such marked improvements in thera- peutic methods that we find certain and tangible evidence thereof in the diminishing fatality of any disease ? Can one mention a single malady which thirty years ago resisted every remedial effort to which the more enlightened science of to-day can offer hopes of recovery? These seem to me perfectly legitimate and fair questions, and, fortunately, in one respect, capable of a scientific reply. I suppose the opinion of the late Claud Bernard, of Paris, would be generally accepted as that of the highest scientific authority on the utility of vivisection in ' practical medicine '; but he tells us that it is hardly worth while to make the inquiry. ' Without doubt,' he confesses, ' our hands are empty to day, although our mouths are full of legitimate promises for the future.' Was Claude Bernard correct in this opinion as to the ' empty hands ' ? If scientific evidence is worth anything, it points to the appalling conclusion that, notwithstanding all the researches of physiology, some of the chief forms of disease exhibit to-day in England a greater fatality than thirty years ago."—" *Vivisection,*" *Lippincott's Magazine*, Aug. 1884, p. 131.

—— The same.

Macilwain.

GEORGE MACILWAIN, F.R.C.S. (the late), a witness before the Royal Commission, 1875 (born 1797 ; died 1882). (A.V.)

" I practised vivisection a little myself, but that was very early indeed. My view is that vivisection is wholly useless, and worse than useless. . . . I only repudiate vivisection as one of the fallacies in medical investigation. . . . I hope I do not yield to any man living in what I feel as to what is due to animals, and to the high nature of investigations ; but I do not wish such considerations to be mixed up with the facts. I would rather it was supposed that I was wonderfully cruel than I would mar the evidence which I believe stands as evidence which is irrefragable.—(Chairman) : What I under- stand you to say is, that you would not tolerate and regulate vivisection, but you would abolish it altogether ?—If you are asking me that as a scientific man. I say most decidedly so. . . . I think it is a demonstrable fallacy."—*Evid. Roy. Com.* (London, 1876), Q. 1853-4-7.

USELESSNESS OF VIVISECTION—Results on Animals no Criterion as to Man.   Savory.

SIR WM. SCOVELL SAVORY, Bart., F.R.C.S., F.R.S. (the late), Ex-President Royal College of Surgeons (born 1826; died 1895). (Doubtful).

" Mr. Savory and Mr. Holmes both urged the objection that experiments conducted on animals afford no criterion as to the results to be expected when similar experiments are made on the human being; and apparently they seemed to imply that this fact detracted from the importance of the observations embodied in the paper."—*From " At the Societies," in the " Medical Press,"* May 19th, 1886.

—— The same.   Sewall.

HENRY SEWALL, B.Sc. ; Ph.D.; Prof. of Physiol. Univ. of Michigan, Ann Arbor, U.S.A. (V.)

" The experiments to be described were carried on by means of the facilities offered at the Marine Laboratory of the Johns Hopkins University during the summer of 1881, at Beaufort, N.C., and again in 1883, on the Chesapeake Bay. . . . Records were made of experiments performed upon more than ninety individuals (sharks and skate). . . . The experiments . . . were performed under unusually favourable anatomical conditions, but it must be confessed that the results obtained are far from forming a solution of the problem investigated."—*Journal of Physiology,* vol. iv. pp. 338, etc.

VERATRIA (*Veratrine*).   Berdoe.

EDWARD BERDOE, M.R.C.S., L.R.C.P.Ed., London. (A.V.)

" Obtained from cevadilla seeds. This is an exceedingly powerful and dangerous alkaloid. Even the minutest quantity brought in contact with the nostrils occasions great and continued irritation, sneezing, and coughing. Injected hypodermically, it causes the most intense pain, as though one were burned with hot needles. Even the fortieth or from that to a twentieth of a grain inserted under the skin causes a tingling which begins in the fingers and toes and extends over the whole body. Yet we know that Kölliker (*Virchow's Archiv*, Bd. x., p. 261) opened the skulls of living frogs and dropped in a solution of the poison, causing 'violent general tetanic convulsions.' Prevost (*Robin's Journal de l'Anatomie*, 1868, p. 209) performed similar experiments, and the Frenchman contradicted the German on every point. We include this drug in our observation, as it illustrates how exceedingly cruel the 'painless hypodermic injections' may be, though they involve no cutting operations whatever. Professor Wood says 'the study of its physiological actions shows that its *rational therapeutical use* (note the distinction) must be limited.'—(*Therapeutics*, p. 169.)"—*The Futility of Experiments with Drugs on Animals*, by Edward Berdoe (London, 1889). p. 42.

VIVISECTION.—Do we affirm that the benefit to mankind is not an adequate or sufficient justification for the infliction of pain on animals? Cobbe.

FRANCES POWER COBBE, Authoress, Hengwrt, Dolgelly, N. Wales. (A.V.)

" You ask us, sir, secondly, ' Do we affirm that the benefit of mankind is not an adequate or sufficient justification for the infliction of pain on animals?' We have two answers to this question.

" Assuming that by vivisection benefits might be obtained for human bodies, we hold that the evil results of the practice on the human mind would more than counterbalance any benefits. The cowardice and pitilessness involved in tying down a dog on a table and slowly mangling its brain, its eyes, its entrails ; the sin committed against love and fidelity themselves when a creature capable of dying of grief on his master's grave is dealt with as a mere parcel of material tissue, ' valuable for purposes of research '—these are basenesses for which no physical advantages would compensate, and the prevalence of such a heart-hardening process among our young men would, we are convinced, detract more from the moral interests of our nation than a thousand cases of recovery from disease would serve those of a lower kind. Even life itself ought not to be saved by such methods, any more than by the cannibalism of the men of the *Mignonette*.

" Our second answer is yet more brief. We do not ' deny that the benefit of man is a sufficient justification for inflicting pain upon animals,' provided that pain is kept within moderate bounds, nor yet to taking life from them in a quick and careful manner. But we do deny the right of man to inflict torture upon brutes, and thus convert their lives from a blessing into a curse. Such torture has been inflicted upon tens of thousands of animals by vivisection; and no legislation that ingenuity can devise will, we believe, suffice to guard against the repetition of it so long as it is sanctioned in any way as a method of research. The use of vivisection—if it have any use—is practically inseparable from abuse."—*Letter in "The Times,"* December 30th, 1884.

VIVISECTION—Senseless and Unscientific.   Lilly.

WILLIAM S. LILLY, LL.M., Barrister-at-Law, Athenæum Club, London. (A.V.)

"It is difficult to conceive of anything more senseless and unscientific than an attempt to interpret morbid states and morbid phenomena by physiological theories, to develop the laws of nature by mutilating the structure of conscient organic beings—every one of them an integral system of most complicated nervous network—to illustrate the modifications which spring up in a disease by processes which are foreign to natural influences. I say nothing of the confusion which also arises from the perfect dissimilarity between the functions and diseases of man and of the lower animals. We live in an era of vivisection. And the voice of reason is as ineffectual against that ghastly shibboleth as it was against the vomiting of the emetic era, the evacuation of the purging era, the depletion of the bleeding era, the poisoning of the mercurial era, and of the iodide of potassium era. Certain it is that the whole race of vivisectors, from the first until now, have not discovered one single agent for the cure of any malady, nor established any therapeutic fact or theory helpful in the smallest degree for the treatment of disease, nor contributed at all to the advance of scientific surgery. Certain it is that some of the most ferocious vivisections upon record—those, for example, of Dr. Bennett and Dr. Rutherford on the biliary secretion of the dog—have issued in mere fallacy and absurdity."—*"The New Naturalism," "Fortnightly Review"* (August, 1885).

VIVISECTION—Useless for Mankind.   Blackwell.

ELIZABETH BLACKWELL, M.D., Hastings. (A.V.)

"In 1849-50, I was a student in Paris, and with the narrow range of thought which marks youth, I was extremely interested in the investigations respecting the liver and gall-bladder,

which Claude Bernard (Majendie's successor) was then carrying on and lecturing upon at the Collège de France and the
Sorbonne. I called upon M. Bernard to ask him where I
could find some work on ' Physiologie Appliquée,' which would
show me how the results of these investigations could be applied
to the benefit of man. M. Bernard received me with the
utmost courtesy, but told me there was no such book written
—the time had not come for the deductions I sought—experimenters were simply accumulating facts. We are still, forty
years later, vainly accumulating facts! This present summer,
Dr. Semmola, 'one of the most brilliant pupils of Claude
Bernard,' lectured in Paris on Bright's disease, which he has
been studying for forty years with unlimited experimentation
on the lower animals, for the purpose of producing in them
artificial inflammation and disease of the kidneys. What is the
result to the human being of all this prolonged and ingenious
suffering inflicted on helpless creatures? Dr. Semmola
insisted upon temperance in eating as well as drinking, and
said that the best way to preserve health was to eat only what
was needed for the nourishment of the body!

* * * * *

"In late discussions in the French Academy of Medicine
relative to chloroform, when Laborde and Franck exhibited
experiments on animals, the distinguished surgeon, Dr. Le
Forte, said, ' None of these experiments give us any instruction
whatever which is useful in practical surgery. Whatever their
scientific interest may be, the deductions from them are in no
way applicable to man.' Again, at another discussion in the
French Academy, M. Verneuil said : ' It is incorrect to say that
laboratory experiments give certainty to medicine and make it
scientific instead of empirical. The fact is that experimentation
has put forth as many errors as truths.'"—*Erroneous Method
in Medical Education. An Address to the Alumnæ of the
Women's Medical College of New York Infirmary, by Dr.
Elizabeth Blackwell* (1891).

VIVISECTORS—Indifference of, to Suffering.   Cobbe.

FRANCES POWER COBBE, Authoress, Hengwrt, Dolgelly, North
Wales. (A.V.)

"Such indifference to suffering as we have imagined in our
hypothetical cases of artists, or sanitary reformers, or cooks,
or sportsmen, would, on the whole, be less monstrous and
anomalous than the passion for vivisection among the men of
science ; and this for two noticeable reasons. In the first place,

artists, sportsmen, and *bon-vivants*, know comparatively little
of the nature and extent of the suffering caused by lacerations
of the living tissues, or the production of morbid conditions,
while the physiologists understand the matter to a nicety, and
have the most perfect acquaintance with every pain which
they cause—nay, the causation of which is often the immediate
object of their ingenious exertions.   As the writer of a letter
in the *Pall Mall Gazette*, bearing the well-known signature of
'Lewis Caroll,' expressed it: 'What can teach the noble
quality of mercy, of sensitiveness to every form of suffering, so
powerfully as the knowledge of what suffering really is?   Can
the man who has once realized by minute study what the nerves
are, what the brain is, and what waves of agony the one can
convey to the other, go forth and wantonly inflict pain on any
sentient being?   A little while ago we should have confidently
replied, " He cannot do it."   In the light of modern revelations
we must sorrowfully confess he can.' "—*The Moral Aspects of
Vivisection*, 6th edit. (London, 1884).

VIVISECTORS—No excuse to say they are good men.—*See*
Good Men.

WANTON VIVISECTION.   Various Authorities.

Mr. P. D. Handyside, M.D., F.R.S.E., being examined,
repudiated "associating" himself with the experiments of Mr.
Hoggan's student days, but acknowledges that he advised him
to make them, and offered him a room.   (Q. 5,972): "   .   .   .
The professors and teachers in the University of Edinburgh
think it their duty to encourage any young man who shows a
certain amount of scientific aptitude to carry out original research, and to embody the original scientific research in the
thesis.   .   .   .?" (Question originally put to Dr. Hoggan, now
put to Professor Handyside.)--" Clearly it is so."

Mr. W. B. A. Scott, M.D., asked (Q. 5,238) : " Have you any
knowledge at all as to whether the practice of vivisection goes on
amongst students of either of these universities ? "--Answered :
" Yes, among the students in their own rooms."

Dr. J. Anthony says (Q. 2,513) that "juveniles" in the
"provinces" experiment; "they tell me candidly what they are
doing, and I am obliged to shake my head occasionally."
(Q. 2,514): " Are these young medical practitioners ?"—" Yes."
(Q. 2,515): " Who, in your judgment, are engaged in vivisection
without any justifiable object, and merely for curiosity ? "—
" Merely from curiosity."   (Animals used were guinea pigs,
kittens, cats, and stray dogs in private houses, anæsthetics not

being used.) (Q. 2,532) : "You stated . . . that within your knowledge medical practitioners in the country were in the habit of performing experiments which you considered cruel and unnecessary?"—"Yes, they have come to my knowledge."—*Evid. Roy. Com.* (London, 1876).

WANTON EXPERIMENTS not   Various Authorities.
performed, according to Drs.
Rutherford and Gamgee.

Professor Rutherford, in answer to question 2,989, says : " I really have had no personal experience of any unnecessary or reckless vivisection on any part of the Continent."

Dr. A. Gamgee, F.R.S., Brackenbury Professor of Physiology at Owens College, stated that he knew several foreign physiologists " pretty intimately," and is then asked—(Q. 5,418) : " Do you not think that a good many of them perform experiments which the English physiologists would mostly regard as needless, and even wanton ?"—"I confess to you I do not believe it."

And yet Dr. Sharpey states (Q. 444) in reference to Majendie's laboratory in Paris:—"I was so utterly repelled by what I witnessed that I never went back again " (explains that the experiments were *painful*, and without any sufficient object), " Majendie made incisions into the skins of rabbits and other creatures to show that the skin is sensitive. Now, surely all the world knows that the skin is sensitive. He put the animals to death finally in a very painful manner."

Dr. Anthony, also speaking of Paris, says (Q. 2,582) : "The men there seem to care no more for the pain of the creature operated upon than if it were so much inorganic matter." In answer to Q. 2,448, the same gentleman stated that the carelessness was also shown as to the end of animals after experimentation. Often they were allowed to simply "crawl" into a corner to die.

Mr. F. Sibson, M.D., says—(Q. 4,739) : "When Majendie was doing these ruthless things, Sir Charles Bell was erring in the opposite direction ; and I believe it was the opposite polarity, induced by the ruthlessness of Majendie, which caused the over-fastidiousness of Sir Charles Bell."

Sir James Paget (Q. 369) says of Majendie, " he seemed really quite indifferent to pain."

In answer to Question 6,374, Mr. G. H. Lewes says : " Yes ; what I wish is that there should be more thoughtful experimenters, and fewer needless experiments."—*Evid. Roy. Com.* (London, 1876).

WOODY NIGHTSHADE (*Solanum Dulcamara*).—Conflict of Experiments on Animals and Human Beings.   Berdoe.

EDWARD BERDOE, M.R.C.S., L.R.C.P.Ed., London. (A.V.)

" The extract of this plant when introduced into the stomach of rabbits causes a remarkable degree of apathy with blunted sensibility.   It reduces the frequency of the pulse and the respiration, and brings on later, convulsions and death.   Dr. John Harley experimented with it on man, without causing any appreciable physiological effect. Whereupon Dr. Stillé *(Therapeutics*, p. 519) makes the following admirable remarks :—' The so-called scientific therapeutists of the present day are disposed to deny any curative virtues to dulcamara, because they are unable to explain those it is alleged to possess, according to their notions of its mode of action.   Such a reason may, in a logical sense, be called impertinent.   The claims of dulcamara rest on the same grounds as those of opium, mercury, and cinchona, the ground of clinical experience.' "

" According to *Woodman and Tidy's Forensic Medicine and Toxicology*, 1st Ed., p. 434, M. Duval gave 180 Woody Nightshade berries as well as four ounces of the extract to dogs without producing any effect, yet death is recorded to have been produced by two berries in a child four years old."—*The Futility of Experiments with Drugs on Animals*, by Edward Berdoe (London, 1889), p. 43.

YELLOW FEVER—INOCULATION FOR.   Moxly.

J. H. S. MOXLY, The Firs, Brentwood, Essex.

" As the first experimentalist to bring to a test the statements, alluded to in your leading article of to-day, as to the supposed discovery in Brazil of a microbe which was the cause of yellow fever, kindly permit me to point out that such statements have no solid basis.   Professor Harrison (of the Government Laboratories, Demerara) and the writer of this letter, having jointly conducted a series of experiments upon the development of yellow fever, became convinced, in 1883, that the statements as to the discovery of a specific yellow fever microbe were premature, and that the system of preventive inoculation introduced by a Brazilian Professor was futile and dangerous.   An account of the experiments on which our conclusions were based, with a statement of the reasons which compelled us to differ absolutely from the supposed discoverer, was published by the Government of the day in the Blue-book (Colonies, 1884), and also, for greater circulation, in separate form as a pamphlet. Soon after the publication of our Report, the Governments of France and of the United States of America sent out Commissioners (experts) to the West Indies to investigate on the spot the claims of the so-called discovery. The Commissioners of the two countries, agreeing with one another in the main, both denied the reality of the discovery, and came in effect to the same conclusions at which we had previously arrived. The cause and origin of yellow fever remain up to the present time unknown, and the 'treatment' of the disease has not yet passed beyond the empiric stage." —*Letter in " The Standard " (London)*, August 20th, 1892.

YELLOW JASMINE (*Gelsemium*). Berdoe.

EDWARD BERDOE, M.R.C.S., L.R.C.P.Ed., London. (A.V.)

" Rabbits and cats, when poisoned by Gelsemium, perform very remarkable backward movements, in which sometimes a complete backward somersault occurs. No corresponding acts have taken place in the fatal cases observed in man. Bartholow says (p. 415) that Ringer and Ott, in an elaborate series of investigations, have confirmed his experimental observations, but he regrets that they were regarded as ' inconclusive ' by Dr. H. C. Wood.

" Dr. Stillé says (p. 676), that ' incalculable mischief ' has been produced by using this and other drugs ' upon no better ground than their power of lowering the pulse and depressing the nervous system.' The experimental school of physiologists look upon the animal organism as merely a complicated machine ; powerless to solve the mystery of being, they ignore it and treat its disturbances of function as they would treat a watch or a steam engine out of order. The stomach is but a superior sort of test tube, the blood vessels mere conduits, and the nerves electric wires, all to be regulated on chemical and mechanical principles ; hence the abundant errors and the irreconcilable confusion which have occupied our attention in these pages. What else could have been expected ? "—*The Futility of Experiments with Drugs on Animals*, by Edward Berdoe (London, 1889), pp. 43, 44.

INDEX TO AUTHORS.

S

T

www.ingramcontent.com/pod-product-compliance
Lightning Source LLC
Chambersburg PA
CBHW030351270326
41926CB00009B/1048